Letters from a Sex Addict

My Life Exposed

Wendy Conquest

Dan Drake

ISBN: 1545306419

ISBN 13: 978-1545306413

Library of Congress Control Number: 2017905936

CreateSpace Independent Publishing Platform

North Charleston, South Carolina

Cover design by Violet Farley

Praise for
Letters from a Sex Addict

"With these fictional yet fact-based letters from sex addicts, Wendy Conquest and Dan Drake show the progression of sex and porn addiction from the addict's perspective, including all of the denial, confusion, and unfettered emotions that sex addicts typically experience. Sex addicts will see themselves in this book, and their betrayed partners will develop a better understanding of what happens in the addict's mind and heart."

- Robert Weiss, LCSW, CSAT-S, author of *Sex Addiction 101: A Basic Guide to Healing from Sex, Porn, and Love Addiction* (and other books)

"In *Letters from a Sex Addict,* Wendy Conquest and Dan Drake skillfully reveal inner reflections of the thinking and feeling of sex addicts at different phases of crisis and recovery. They creatively weave the letters from addicts with practical advice to guide the reader toward understanding and hope. Reading like both a personal journal and self-help book, *Letters from a Sex Addict* is sure to become a critical reference book for clinicians as well as for the addict and partner looking for direction."

- Kenneth M. Adams, Ph.D., CSAT-S, author of *Silently Seduced* and *When He's Married to Mom*

"Authors Drake and Conquest do an incredible job of bring the voice of sex addiction to life. The letters provided offer a realistic glimpse into the life of the addict and are a profound demonstration of the progression of the disease over time. This text will provide insight to addicts and family members alike, and is a great contribution to the field."

- Stefanie Carnes, IITAP President, author of numerous publications including *Facing Heartbreak*

"In Letters, the authors provide a realistic, first-person and inside-out reveal of the sex addict's world of shame and secrets. This unique perspective is a necessary read for those struggling with or affected by sexual addiction and who want to make sense of the addict's denial, blame or betrayal."

- Debra L. Kaplan, MA, MBA, LPC, CSAT-S, author of *For Love and Money: Exploring Sexual & Financial Betrayal in Relationship*

"This book does a great job of articulating the sex addiction experience from a client's perspective. For the individual who is struggling with their sexual behaviors, *Letters from a Sex Addict* provides different perspectives from which people can relate. An easy read, this book illustrates the different thought process, positive and negative, often experienced during the different stages of recovery."

- Todd Love, PsyD, JD, LPC, author specializing in problematic sexual behaviors

"*Letters from a Sex Addict* is a must read for all couples facing the painful journey of sexual addiction recovery. The letters capture the reality of the gut wrenching impact that sex addiction has on the addict, partner, and relationship. By understanding the inner world of the sex addict, and normalizing the wild, emotional roller coaster ride during the various phases of recovery, the letters provide hope and a path for healing and mature love to grow."

- Dorit Reichental, MA MFTi, ASAT, CPC, relational trauma expert and couples coach

"In *Letters from a Sex* Addict, authors and therapists Wendy Conquest and Dan Drake combine their clinical experience in sharing a supportive resource for sex addicts and their hurting partners. *Letters from a Sex Addict* addresses a wide range of issues faced by people in recovery and will provide helpful guidance for those individuals who are moving through the healing process as well as the therapists who support them."

- Mari Lee, LMFT, CSAT-S, author of *Facing Heartbreak: Steps to Recovery for Partners of Sex Addicts* and *The Creative Clinician: Exercises and Activities for Clients and Group Therapy*, clinical director of Growth Counseling Services, Glendora, California and founder of the Counselor's Coach

"Wendy and Dan's book, *Letters from a Sex Addict*, takes the reader into the raw experience and reflections of people (a person) caught by–and recovering from–the grips of sex addiction. This book can be a "safe" meeting space for both the addict and the partner, where each can enter the experiences common to the addict. One of the main ingredients of recovery for both the addict and their partners is that of empathy. To hear real stories and reflections puts flesh on the bones of the psychological theory, making it less academic and more real. I will recommend this book to all my clients going through the pain and suffering related to sex addiction."

- Sam Alibrando, PhD, clinical psychologist and author of *Follow the Yellow Brick Road: How to Change for the Better When Life Gives You Its Worst* and *The Three Dimensions of Emotion: Finding the Balance of Power, Heart and Mindfulness*

"'Letters from a Sex Addict,' is a must-read for anyone who has ever struggled with sexual issues in their lives. Instead of the typical clinical or self-help book, it doesn't preach at you. Or tell you how to fix your deep inner struggles in 10 or 12 easy steps. Instead, you hear the visceral and real words of men and women caught in the death grip of the addictive process. It also presents the clarion cry of individuals how have won the struggle. Again it is a must read for the first step in the long journey to wholeness and health. After thirty years of counseling addicts and leading groups, nothing gives folks hope like hearing the honest words of fellow warriors."

- Dr. Ted Roberts PSAP-S, founder of Pure Desire Ministries International

"Finally a book that cracks the door open to places we dare to tread. Having been the wife of a sex addict who lived with pornography, affairs and prostitutes; what I couldn't fathom is what he was thinking? These *soul-slicing* letters not only answered questions I've had for decades, but helped me see two things – we're painfully human *AND* I'm not alone."

-   Sheri Keffer, PhD, MFT, CCPS, CSAT-C,
    Certified Clinical Partner Specialist and co-host of
    New Life Live Radio and TV

"*Letters from a Sex Addict* is an opportunity for sex addicts in any state of their recovery to appreciate that they are not alone in their thinking, their behavior or their recovery. This is a must read for a sex addict as it will enlighten him and provide much gratitude for the progress he has made.

The authors have compiled information from their clients that will assist readers in making sense of sexual addiction and the partner trauma that occurs from it. *Letters from a Sex Addict* is both profoundly personal and clinically illuminating making it a must read for clinicians as well.

It is a great reminder of the stages of sexual addiction recovery."

-   Carol Juergensen Sheets, LCSW, PCC, CSAT, author
    of numerous publications and podcasts, radio show
    host, and Certified Personal Life and Executive
    Coach

"Letters from a Sex Addict is a bold, new venture into the process of healing sex addiction. In a painfully real way Conquest and Drake have compiled summaries of the vast number of conversations I've witnessed in my 30 years of working in this field. Not only do they explore the struggle and the natural ambivalence about the early process painfully well, they also have compiled a beautiful experience of the journey through healing to recovery, with all its amazement and uncertainty. Even before reading the Appendix describing the grief process, I read into the letters all the many stages of healing the losses of addiction and recovery. Their gentle insistence on viewing this process through the lenses of denial, bargaining, protest (anger) is essential in exposing and grasping the sadness and necessary acceptance that is not only necessary, but also inherent in the healing process. Reading through the section 'Moving Forward' was a touching reminder of the goal of the work I do in this field. This will be on the 'Must Read' list for those hoping to find long-lasting peace and recovery."

- James "Jes" Montgomery, MD, CSAT-S, addiction and sexuality expert

To all affected by sex or pornography addiction,
and to those who are still unsure

TABLE OF CONTENTS

Part Two – Unraveling   37

Part Three – Putting Things Together   63

Foreword

I'm so glad this book was written and am grateful for the opportunity to recommend it to you!

Sex addiction. Just these two words can create a wide variety of responses: confusion, disbelief, anger, fear, shame, or a punch line for a bad joke. As a society, we still do not even agree that "sex addiction" is a real condition or a struggle. Those of us in the mental health/addiction fields are still arguing over words or terms to describe out of control and destructive sexual behaviors.

However, those who have directly experienced the impact and consequences of out of control, compulsive sexual behaviors that produce destruction and distress, know all too well that this "thing" or condition exists. They've lived it.

For the person who has the out of control sexual behaviors (we use the words *sex addiction*- its so much shorter and describes what it is like), the reality of feeling obsessed with and controlled by cycles of sexual acting out is an every day experience. The shame, the fear, the attempts to control, and the falling back into the behaviors are real. This is the life of an addict prior to recovery.

For loved ones- especially the intimate partner or spouse of the addict- the destruction is equally as real. For the partner, it is typical for them to be unaware of the sexual secrets and acting out for years. They become suddenly aware and blindsided by the reality of the addiction when the secret is broken and evidence is discovered. For the partner, this "D-day" of discovery is one that can be shattering, traumatic, devastating, confusing, and terrifying

1

(Steffens, 2005). The destruction is immediate and on going. Its like an earthquake that feels like it will never end.

Since the 1970s and 1980s when brave men and women started speaking out about this disorder and its destruction, the profession of treating sex addiction has grown and improved. Hope and recovery became a possibility. However, it is really only in the past decade that real focus has been placed on the needs of the intimate partner or spouse.

In the early days of this profession, the partner or spouse was conceptualized as someone with their own disorder or addiction and all partners were treated the same. The partner (the profession used words like "co-dependent" or "co-addict") required assistance. Treatment methods were focused on helping the out of control partner or "co-addict" SO THAT the treatment process of the person with the addiction would go more smoothly. The addict was often protected from the intensity of the partner, by a process that communicated that the partner was "as sick as" the addict. The partner or "co-addict" then was to focus on his or her own recovery so that the addict could focus on theirs. We've come to understand that model of treatment as "addict-centric"- the partner was given assistance in order to support the treatment of the addict.

As a profession, many of us have been moving into a more "partner-sensitive" model of treatment and support, where the needs and experiences of the partner are seen as just as needed and important as the needs of the addict. We are learning that if we provide real support to a traumatized partner and help the addict understand the experiences of the partner in response to the betrayal of sexual addiction,

2

the whole system does better. There is more hope for recovery for everyone.

There are many resources available that describe sex addiction and recovery. There are a growing number of resources that describe the impact of sex addiction on the partner and trauma recovery since the publication of *Your Sexually Addicted Spouse: How Partners Can Cope and Heal* (Steffens & Means) in 2009. There have not been resources that were written to help get inside the experiences of the partners or addicts until now. Wendy Conquest's *Letters to a Sex Addict- The Journey Through Grief and Betrayal* (2013) was a first to present the struggle and pain of partners of addicts through "first person" writings. These letters provided windows into the hearts and lives of partners throughout the discovery, trauma, and healing journey.

Now, Wendy and Marriage and Family Therapist Dan Drake have added to this wonderful resource by writing *Letters from a Sex Addict*.

The letters in this book provide a look into the thought processes, emotions, shame, and experiences of those struggling with sexual addiction and discovery and recovery. The letters are raw and real. And the letters can provide hope.

I so appreciate this book. For partners, the letters can help them "see inside" the mind of the one they love; to see the confusion, the distorted thinking, the fear and the humanity of the addict. For anyone with this addiction, the letters can offer the knowledge that they are not alone, that others share their struggle, and that others have gone before them on the recovery journey. There is hope.

I also love this *book series* because it helps those in relationships ravaged by sexual addiction find connection, empathy, and the ability to imagine a way forward. These books can help two wounded people begin to understand each other. **Rather than contributing to isolating both partners (as we've too often experienced in this field), these books can become important tools to bridge the gap caused by sexual addiction and betrayal.**

Letters From a Sex Addict -- this collection of "letters" from sex addicts -- is powerful and will become a very important recovery resource for all those impacted by out of control sexual behaviors or sex addiction. The authors do a masterful job of laying out the process of recovery for the sex addict who is in relationship, along with clearly describing the traumatic impact on the addict and the spouse or partner after sexual secrets are discovered. Through this collection of writings, they illustrate the process of recovery: the shock and trauma of discovery, to moving out from denial, to ambivalence and fear, to decision and determination, to "getting it" and then on to moving beyond addiction. Not only does this book provide accurate descriptions of the difficult work and grief and trauma implicit in addiction recovery, it also imparts wisdom and hope to the reader, as the process of recovery unfolds in each chapter.

I encourage you to use this book as part of your own recovery process; this is appropriate for the person with the addictive behaviors <u>and</u> for the partner/spouse. Use the questions at the end of each section to dig deeper into your own thoughts, feelings, and experiences.

Recovery is a journey no one can take alone. This book can be one of your companions as you seek to find the way individually and together in recovery.

Barbara Steffens PhD LPCC, CCPS
Co-author *Your Sexually Addicted Spouse: How Partners Can Cope and Heal* (Steffens & Means, 2009).
President of the Board, *The Association of Partners of Sex Addicts Trauma Specialists.*

Introduction

Sex addiction. Porn addict. These are not pretty words or great labels to associate ourselves with. But at the end of the day, it doesn't matter what we call it. The question is, do you want to stop a pattern of sexual or sexualized behavior? Do you want to improve your life? Do you want to stop hurting others? Do you want to stop hurting yourself? If you are the partner or family member affected by a loved one's sexual behaviors, do you want to understand what has happened?

Of all things we can become addicted to, sex often has the most damaging impact on others. Partners will say they were shocked and hurt when they found out their loved one was an alcoholic. When they discovered they had a drug addiction, they would have gladly gone back to their being an alcoholic. When the love of their life confessed to being a sex addict, they yearned for the addiction to "only" be drugs.

As a society we condone sex addiction. We tell each other that "everyone watches porn," and "strippers really like what they do, she told me so." The belief that "sex sells" has become an excuse for more outlandish sexual depictions of girls and women. We now know that the human brain seeks novelty and thus the advertising and marketing campaigns seek more inventive ways to grab our attention, which has created more violent and perverse images. One problem with this is our young people are convinced that this is the way men and women should look and behave. Our ability to recognize what healthy sexuality looks and feels like has become obscured and polluted. When a twenty-four-year-old man is confused because his girlfriend is surprised that he hasn't asked to have anal sex, something is terribly wrong.

But we've digressed. This book is about the progression of sex and porn addiction from the addict's perspective. We have worked with thousands of men and women in all the stages of recovery. Often it is the wife or girlfriend, husband or lover who insists on assessment and treatment, which gets the addicted person in our therapy offices. Many times the couple comes in seeking help for the relationship. We consistently see a lot of confusion and desperation. Both the person who has been sexually acting out and the partner who has found out her loved one has a secret life are in shock. They both have ideas and expectations about how this journey will go. This book is meant to provide an inside look at the addict's world. We've written across a spectrum of different responses to the addiction: from some in great denial, to some wanting help but not quite ready, to some wholeheartedly jumping into recovery.

You will see the format is in letter form. Letters are a personal communication between two people. Communication, when living together, is usually verbal, or in short texts or e-mails. Important, emotional, thought-through verbiage elicits a hand-written letter. This is the spirit we wished to convey. In addition, we now know that the partner undergoes shock and trauma and that her brain becomes compromised. Normal reading abilities and information retention are lessened so shorter pieces of writing are easier to absorb.

There are descriptions of the different reactions of the addict throughout the book. The healing process is usually challenging and fraught with setbacks, hope, fear, disappointment, and disillusionment. We wanted to portray a realistic presentation. We wanted the addict to be able to point to where he is at in his recovery and know he can succeed. We wanted the spouse to be able to have a map at the end of each chapter; what is healthy and unhealthy behavior in relation to what her husband is saying and doing, to provide an anchor of sanity. With that said, please understand that words alone do not create safety or trust in the relationship. We have found that constant and continual behavioral change of the addict is crucial.

The letters in this book track the journey of men and women recovering from sex addiction. We've broken this journey up into different stages, with explanations at the beginning of each section, and questions for you to consider at the end of each chapter. If you are in recovery from sexual addiction, you may choose to read this as part of your work with a sponsor or therapist. You may find it helpful to share in a group or meeting. If you are a partner of someone in recovery from sex addiction, you may find it helpful to read these letters to better understand the mindset of typical addicts in different phases of the process. We recommend that you find a trusted person or group to talk with you about what you are reading. Most of all, we hope this book helps you to better understand the world of sexual addiction, knowing that there IS a path, and the road to recovery is possible. We see people step onto this journey every day. We see people committed to this process recover and heal. We wish the same for you.

These letters are a fictional version of past and present experiences of our patients. The content herein is not any individual's life story but a composite from hundreds of clients the authors have treated. We will frequently use masculine pronouns (e.g., he, his, him) to represent the sex addict, and feminine pronouns (e.g., she, hers, her) to represent the partner of the sex addict. We recognize that though many addicts are male and their partners are female, addicts can be male or female and can be single or in a same-sex relationship.

What is Sex Addiction?
The Sex Addiction Journey

I keep hearing from family, friends, and social media that "sex addiction" is a nice excuse for letting jerks off the hook for doing bad things. Maybe they're right. I've definitely done some bad things. I've harmed my wife beyond anything I can possibly imagine. When my story became public I shamed my family and community. I even got kicked out of my church. I get it. I probably would've done the same thing were I not the one going through this. Yet I thought I'd write a bit more about what sex addiction means to me. I can't say this is everyone's story, but I've been to enough meetings and heard enough "first steps" to know that I'm not alone here. I'm not writing this to justify my behaviors either: I DID do that in the past, but I now know that I'm 100% responsible for all my actions. I hope in writing this letter that I can explain to others what sex addiction is. I want to spare other people and their families from the pain that I've put myself and my whole world through.

So what is sex addiction? I've heard a lot of definitions of sex addiction, but what it is to me is an intense hunger for intimacy and a terror of it at the same time. It may seem strange, but I DO love my wife. I would be devastated if she left me. She's the best thing that's ever happened to me. I've learned, though, because of my early abuse and neglect growing up, that relying on others wasn't safe for me. I learned that I could feel better for just a little bit when I masturbated. I didn't know how to talk to anyone about this, and so what started as something that made me feel better, over the years became a secret place of shame that ruled my life. I did everything to hide my behaviors from my friends, family, and I hid the real damage of what I was doing even from myself. I wanted to be close to my wife, but I hid from her instead. I turned to others to fill me up. Of course this was only fleeting, and I had to get more and more of the "fix" to have the same impact on me. That's when what started as a way of coping began ruling my life. I've learned that I traded *intimacy* for *intensity*. I know now that what I REALLY wanted was to know and be known at the depths of my soul. But I shied away from that vulnerability and found excitement in secret sexual experiences instead.

It seems easier to talk about alcohol or drugs, and how these can become addicting. Most of us know that we can get addicted to chemicals. Over time we need more and more of the substance to get the same "high" and our behaviors start to escalate. We often may try to stop the behaviors (for me I tried over and over. "This time will be the last time," I told myself. I probably swore that hundreds of times, yet it was never the last time). Inevitably, drained of my fix and not knowing how to deal with my feelings, I'd turn back to the only source of comfort I knew – sex. Even though I knew it was empty, part of my brain needed more and more. I became preoccupied, obsessed about when I would be "acting out." It took over my work and home life, and this led to many negative consequences. Yet, often these results weren't enough to keep me from going back. It wasn't until my wife finally discovered me, confronted me, and gave me an ultimatum that I woke up. That was the beginning of my journey of recovery. And though it hasn't been perfect, the fog has been lifted, and I can now more clearly see the insanity that I was in when in my addiction.

I know there will still be plenty of people who use the label of sex addict as an excuse, or even to stay in shame. But I know that just as we can get addicted to chemicals like alcohol, nicotine, or opiates, we can also get addicted to experiences, like gambling, shopping, eating, and sex. Unfortunately, I've seen how personal this addiction is. It cuts to the core of my relationship and has hurt my wife tremendously. I would give anything to be "just" a drug addict, but this is where I am. What I can do is to continue my recovery, continue growing, and continue to be a source of healing for myself, my wife, my family, and my community.

Part One:

In the Dark

Sexual addiction frequently takes many years to develop. After the addiction progresses, many years can transpire before an individual gets into recovery. During these years, we often find a pattern of lies, deception, distortions, and secrecy that the addict employs with those in his life. These patterns may be conscious or unconscious, but they serve to keep his secret sexual behaviors hidden from others.

Small or large life experiences start to occur to reveal the addiction. This may include nearly being caught, a friend commenting on behaviors, a partner challenging words or actions. Because the sexual compulsivity has become part of a pattern, the addict usually has little or no awareness that anything is wrong or amiss. Further along in recovery, we find that there was an underlying sense that life was not right. However, at this stage this quickly gets dismissed.

The real challenge occurs when the addict tries to convince himself that he can stop at any time, attempts to, and then goes back to the acting out. This is usually the first indication that there's a problem. The addict mind, however, is crafty at fooling everyone, including itself, such as; "I had myself convinced that what I was doing was no big deal", and "It's what I had learned from my dad and my dad's dad so how could it be wrong?", and "It's what everyone else was doing so I thought it was okay." These statements are indicative of the addict's distorted perspective.

Please note that the letters in this section are pre-recovery. They are in the book so that addicts can resonate with their denial and

17

partners can hear the delusion of someone in active addiction starting to question.

Before getting into recovery, addicts can say and do some pretty awful things. When they look back on this time after significant recovery, they can see how distorted their thinking was, and how much in the "fog" they were. At the time, though, the escalation of their behaviors, or the traumatic impact of their actions on those around them is lost. They may withdraw, lie, gaslight, abuse, become aggressive, or put loved ones in physical danger due to their reckless actions. Sadly though, at this point, few can see what they're really doing.

For partners...*if you are hearing your loved one say these things, this is the addict talking. Please do not take this in as true or rational or even what he really feels and believes. You may find yourself feeling crazy or confused by your partner's behaviors. You may feel that something is wrong but you can't quite put your finger on it. You may have even discovered part of your partner's behaviors, only to have them easily explained or turned on you. Please know that you are not alone, and find a therapist who specializes in sex addiction who can help you understand what may be happening in your relationship.*

For addicts...*if you agree with the letters in this section, you are still in denial about what is happening to you. We encourage you to get help from a counselor or therapist that can assess for sex or porn addiction, go to a sex addiction 12-step group, and know this is not how you need to continue to live.*

So Weird – San Diego, California

The other day a guy in my unit said he stopped watching porn. He said it wasn't right for his marriage; that it takes away from his wife. So weird. Doesn't everyone watch porn?

A Little Scary – Charleston, South Carolina

I keep a journal. And the other day I thought I would go back and read some. My friends are commenting that I am always with a guy and never take time out for me or just to be with my friends. I don't think that's right! I think I've been a true friend to other girls through the years.

And then I started reading my old diaries. One day I am upbeat and confident. I have plans for my life with goals and a clear vision. The next day I am obsessed that Tom or John or Sam hasn't called or texted. I feel hopeless. I can't concentrate on my work. I don't feel good about myself. I write "I'm depressed." I'm thinking I'm not pretty enough or wasn't good enough in bed. As soon as the guy does call or e-mail, I'm on Cloud 9 again. It's almost like I'm two different people. It's a little scary.

PORN – New York, New York

Another late night porn spree leaves me exhausted at work yet again today. This seems to be my night-time ritual more often than not these days. But what does it matter? You hardly seem to notice me anymore. You're busy with work, with the kids. What room is there for me? I haven't bothered you for sex in over two years. I suppose you *have* initiated sex, or at least you used to. But we both know you don't *really* want it.

Truth is, I don't really want sex. I blame you for our lack of sex, but most of all I find myself counting down the hours until you go to bed. I sometimes conjure ways of getting you to sleep earlier so that I can spend my own time, alone with my computer. Even writing this gets me thinking about what I will find tonight. Whatever I discover has to be better than our boring existence right now. What are we even doing??? At least porn will always be there, ready for me when I'm interested. Available when you aren't. Comforting when you don't care. Any refuge from this depressing life.

Just a few more hours . . .

I'm a (Good) Liar – Boston, Massachusetts

Yesterday you asked me what I had for lunch the other day during my business meeting. I told you that I had a salad. But you know, I really had a steak. Here's the funny thing: I didn't even think twice about lying to you about having the steak. I'm not really sure why I lied, but it was the first time I thought about how much I stretch the truth.

Of course there are the big things that I don't want you to know. You can't know about my secret safes and the arrangement website I'm on. That's obvious. I'm pretty good about covering my tracks there.

But why lie about steak?!? That one still blows my mind. As I work to keep all the women, money, scheduling, accounts, and stories straight I'm beginning to wonder if *I* even know which way is up anymore...

What is Happening to Me?!? – Ajo, Arizona

I think I'm going crazy......... Every time I tell myself "this is the last time," I really believe it. But you know what? For every "last time" there comes yet another time. This is crazy - how hard is it to *not* pick up prostitutes??? If I hate myself every time afterward, why do I keep going back again and again?

I know I can never tell you about this - this is my dirty little secret. But I hate myself for it. I just want to stop. I SWEAR, this is the last time. It HAS to be.

feeling this of lack of sex and inability to invalidate

JUST ONE LAST TIME – Columbus, Ohio

The New Year is fast approaching - just three more days. It's no surprise what my biggest New Year's resolution is this year. Of course I can't tell you this, but on January 1st I'm going to deactivate all my secret accounts and destroy everything I've saved on my hard drives. I really feel different this time. I've tried this before, but something feels different this time. I've got a new resolve.

I'm going to take the next few days to sift through everything I've collected. I really think that'll help me let it go. Maybe I'll even test my resolve by opening up some of those accounts. They don't have the same hold on me like they've had in the past. How free I feel!

Or maybe I'll just give it one last hurrah. Mardi Gras comes before Lent, right? Ok, just this one last time. I do have three more days after all.

HASSLED – Santa Fe, New Mexico

Could you PLEASE just leave me alone? I'm
stressed! I am working my ass off, as we
agreed, so that you can stay home with the
kids. I have obligations at church, and you
want me to be more involved with parenting.
THEN you are on me for not helping with the
house! I thought that would be something
YOU would do since you're home all the time.
SO WHAT if I watch porn sometimes! It's not
like I'm getting laid anytime soon anyway.
Every time I approach you, you're busy or too
tired or whatever. Can you please just leave
me alone to do what I want in my all-too-little
spare time?

Finally I know. – Seattle, Washington

I was in the coffee shop and saw a flyer for Sex and Love Addicts Anonymous. I had never heard of this before. Alcoholics Anonymous, yes. This, no. I was intrigued and something told me I should go. So I did.

Awkward walking into a room like that. I tried not to think of what this meant or who might be there. I just went. And then people starting talking about how they couldn't be alone or had to be in a relationship. Some said they mixed up sex with love, or love with sex. Nearly every person had a story that in some way had a piece of my past in it. All my secrets, they shared openly. Things I dared not share with anyone, they talked of with no shame. Years I've been trying to connect with people on this level and have never been able to. Why, in this room, was it so easy with so many?

They used words foreign to me like "sponsor" and "step work" and "bottom lines." I am skeptical of organized anything, but I am going to go back. There is something there that gives me hope. There seems to be a knowledge there that I haven't heard before.

Could I be *addicted* to something I have thought was exactly the way I should act to find joy and happiness?

Gone – Rochester, New York

You went to visit your mother...again.
Fuck you. It's my birthday and you decide
your mother is more important than me.
FUCK YOU. I can't think straight at work.
Everyone is asking what I'm doing this
weekend. Should I go out? And where am
I supposed to go? What am I supposed to
do? Fuck you, fuck you, fuck you.

There's this cute guy at work who just
started. I like him! Maybe he's not doing
anything this weekend. I didn't see a
wedding ring. Oh, but I wear a wedding
ring. Well, a friendly drink wouldn't hurt
anything. Why not? It'll be fun. And I
won't feel as bad about you being gone. I
wonder if he's around today. I'm feeling
better already!

Never Again – Portland, Maine

I'm writing this to myself. I am horrified at what happened today. I crossed a line that I said I would never cross. I'm not even sure how it happened. One minute we are talking – the next thing I know our clothes are off. I just recall….the RUSH!

But now what? Well I just need to make sure that never happens again. And I don't tell anyone and no one needs to know. Done. Over. Never again.

I DON'T WANT TO HURT YOU – St. Louis, Missouri

I am writing this letter not knowing if I will give it to you. I did it again. It's been years. And then I got a text. Simple enough text from her. I thought it was over. I told you it was over. And then I got the text. Why did she have to contact me again? It was my birthday and you were on a business trip and she was reaching out I guess, friendly, I guess, and I knew I shouldn't text back, I knew I just needed to delete the text and forget about it and...I texted back.

God, why did I text back? I can't even answer that now. I feel terrible. I so don't want to keep hurting you. And I don't know why I do it. I don't know why I am so weak. You said that the last time, that I'm weak and heartless, wanting to cause you pain, but I don't! I LOVE YOU! I love you.

You Don't Give Me Enough Credit – Dallas, Texas

I'm smarter than you are. Of course I'd never say
that to your face (I'm no fool). But those are the
facts. I can make you believe whatever I want you
to believe.

- That pile of cash you discovered? Well,
  obviously I saved it to get you a nice present but
  didn't want you to be able to spoil the surprise by
  looking in our bank account. But since you're so
  inconsiderate to snoop through my stuff, I guess
  you won't be getting that present.
- All of these business trips I've been on
  lately? I'm doing quite well for myself, and after
  all – who do you think pays the bills for you to
  have such a nice lifestyle?
- That strange number you found in my phone? I
  don't have any idea who that was! You know
  how crazy people can get access to your
  phone! Why are YOU so suspicious?! You act
  like you've got something to hide.

And so on . . . You know I carry a lot of weight in
this town. I didn't get here for no reason, after
all. You have everything you could ask for. You
know you wouldn't have it any other way.

I'm Bored – San Luis Obispo, California

I know you're perfectly happy to have sex
in the missionary position for the rest of
your life, but here's the deal: I'm not a
missionary. We're in a rut. Vanilla sex is
so....vanilla. You're boring.

If I want to spice things up a little bit to
get what I need out of this relationship,
what's the big deal? I always come home
to you and the kids. If you're not going to
meet my needs, I have to get them met
elsewhere.

I don't see you changing anytime soon, so
I've got to do what I've got to do. I know
you don't understand it, since you're
content to live out your boring white
picket fence life. But I'm a man and I have
needs.

There is Nothing Wrong with Me – Mesa, Arizona

You know I'm kind of tired of you harping on me all the time. "You don't do the dishes." "When are you going to play with the kids more?" Now that we're in this couples counseling it's "When are you going to *attune* to them." Like I even know what that word means!

I work, and I work hard, to try and give you everything you want. Now, NOW you're complaining about my watching porn! Are you kidding me?

So here's the deal. When you start dressing sexier, and maybe having dinner ready when I get home, then I'll stop watching porn.

Wired –Daytona Beach, Florida

I'm a wreck. I have all this work to do and no time
to get things finished. I HATE my job, and there's
no way out. The other guys hate me, they are all
jealous, I think. And I so want to move, but you
don't want to. If only we could move, then I think I
could have the career I've always wanted.

My dad called today and was wondering how we
were doing in that way he has of implying that I am
not doing the right thing by you and the kids. I
don't know what to say to him anymore because I
can never live up to his expectations. NEVER!

I'm stuck and stressed and I can't tell you. You will
say, "Don't worry it'll be all right." Really? Well
who's going to straighten it all out? Me, right? Me
and only me.

I need a break. I'm just going to go on the
computer so I can relax because I just can't sleep
and I have to get to sleep because I'm behind on
that report due. And if I just so happen to watch
some porn, so what? I deserve it.

In the Dark Questions:

For Addicts:

- *What feelings or reactions did you have when reading these letters?*
- *Were there any letters that were particularly difficult for you to read? Which one(s)?*
- *Looking at your own recovery journey, what strategies of lying, deception, abuse, manipulation, withdrawal, etc. have you used in your relationship(s)?*
- *Are there any of these strategies that you still use today? If so, which ones?*
- *After answering these questions, please re-read the letters again. Read them with an open mind, looking for areas of commonality with your own story. Be as open as possible, and as honest with yourself as you possibly can – that's how we heal. Write down any new insights you take away after re-reading the letters.*
- *What new insights have you gained from reading these letters? What do you need to take with you to a trusted guide (therapist, sponsor, close safe friend, mentor, etc.) for further processing?*
- *Make sure to do something healthy for yourself today. See appendix 1 and 2 for healthy self-*

care activities you can do.

For Partners:

- *What feelings or reactions did you have when reading these letters?*
- *Do any of these letters resonate with you more than others? If so, which one(s) and which part(s)?*
- *Have you experienced any of these patterns of lying, deception, abuse, manipulation, withdrawal, etc. that were described in these letters? Please describe.*
- *In the beginning of the recovery process from sexual addiction, it is common for partners to be in the dark as to the nature of the problem and/or to be blamed for the problem. Have you experienced this? If so, how?*
- *What insights have you gained from reading these letters? What do you need to take with you to a trusted guide (therapist, sponsor, close safe friend, mentor, etc.) for further processing?*
- *Make sure to do something healthy for yourself today. See appendix 1 and 2 for healthy self-care activities you can do.*

PART TWO:
UNRAVELING

Sex addiction is birthed, grows, and festers through secrecy and shame. Most sex addicts at their core do not like themselves. They carry negative beliefs about themselves, such as; "I am unlovable," "I'm not enough," "I'm unworthy," "I am a fraud," "I'm a failure," etc. Though the world around them may see a charming, funny, successful, and larger-than-life man, sex addicts feel small, less-than, inadequate, or weak. They hide their more vulnerable selves from their loved ones and sometimes, even from themselves. Sex addicts fight with every ounce of their being to not have these core beliefs exposed, for if they are discovered, they fear they will be discarded.

Unfortunately, there are major ramifications to carrying such a split between the façade the world sees and the dark interior that the sex addict feels. As the negative core of an addict festers, so does the need to present himself even "better" on the outside. He polishes a shiny exterior, while isolating himself and others from his true self. This creates a divide between public self and secret self. He will continue to look good, even though he feels bad. Addictive behaviors are a way of compensating for this negative core – to fill the dark emptiness with something that will make him feel better. Yet turning to a prostitute, to pornography, or to another relationship proves a temporary fix. The fuel supply he receives externally only lasts momentarily, and he finds himself now filled with more shame to add to the emptiness.

This is the typical trajectory of sex addiction; growing in power over time. Most sex addicts want more than anything to maintain their relationships with their partners, friends, and family, but at some point the addiction envelops them.

Holding so much shame, they become enslaved by the very behaviors that they turned to in order to cope. Yet there comes a breaking point, where the secret can no longer be held.

Tragically, it is typically the partner of a sex addict who discovers the illicit behaviors, often with no warning. She is blindsided by reading a text message on her partner's phone, discovering web pages on a computer, or being told by a friend, family member, or even a law enforcement officer. The secret is exposed and her world shatters.

This marks a crisis point for most individuals and couples. What was will never be the same again. The following section details this phase of the journey, when the hidden world of a sex addict is found out. When he is first discovered, there is the feeling of shock, disbelief, sometimes terror and usually relief. And in the midst of having the secret life revealed, he says some pretty crazy things. They don't sound strange to the addict. He tries to make sense why he lied, cheated, manipulated his loved one to make sure they didn't find out. The letters that follow show how distorted the thinking became.

For partners…*if you are hearing your loved one say these things, this is the addict talking. Please do not take this in as true or rational or even what he really feels and believes. If he continues to work his recovery, these types of words and actions will dissipate over time.*

For addicts…if you agree with the letters in this section, you are starting to realize that something is very wrong. You may be wrestling with whether the "label" of sex addiction fits or not. Calling yourself an addict can be threatening and shaming; however, if behaviors have gotten that out of control, we find it easier to admit the chaos we are now experiencing rather than try and fight any name given to it. This is hard work and we want to encourage you to not give up.

Busted – Cincinnati, Ohio

I know I can never share this letter with you . . . You just wouldn't understand. Here's the honest truth - I'm glad you caught me looking at porn. I mean, I'm not GLAD about it - those few seconds have turned our life inside out. But I'm relieved. I feel like a huge weight has been lifted off my chest.

Maybe that's why I've been getting careless lately - leaving screens open, looking at porn when you're just in the other room, not covering my tracks in the same way I used to. I don't think I could've ever told you about what I was doing. But now that you caught me I feel lighter. With my dirty secret exposed I don't have anything to hide. I hate that it blew up my life, but thank God I don't have to hold that secret anymore.

I'm NOT – Grand Rapids, Michigan

Hey, I get it that you think I'm some sort of weird pervert but I'm not! I had that thing with that chick at the office and it's over. So you need to stop hassling me about it and we need to move on. It's your constantly trying to control me that's driving me crazy! And I don't think we need therapy or counseling or anything like that. We're just wasting our money when we could be using it for something really important. If you want I can help more with the house or something. Why don't we go out and just forget about all this?! I'll buy the tequila! :)

I Had To Tell You – Atlanta, Georgia

I…um…I need to tell you something.

First, I'm sorry.

I've had multiple affairs since we got married, some last for a week or a month, there are others that have been a couple of years. I don't know what's happened to me or what's wrong with me. All I know is that I am really screwed up.

I don't want you to be mad. I don't want you to think this is your fault. I don't know what this is except that it's wrong and I can't seem to stop.
I had to tell you. I'm so sorry.

No one understands – Santa Barbara, California

You tricked me. All your awful behavior made me go outside our marriage to seek comfort and kindness. The house had to be perfect. The kids had to be quiet. You wouldn't let me work. We had to go to synagogue. There was no discussion or communication about what I might want or need. It had to be your way...always.

I couldn't take it anymore. And there was the nice guy at the grocery store. He smiled at me. He told me I was pretty. He noticed me, saw when I had my hair up or down. And he would hover over my hand when I bought stamps. It sounds stupid now. I was dying and I couldn't tell you.

And now you and everyone has labeled me a sex addict. Or a love addict. Or both. I don't want to be called that. No one understands. I just want to be left alone.

It Takes Two – Tampa, Florida

My sponsor told me not to say anything about this, but how can I NOT? I'm SICK of this. All the responsibility gets put on me. Somehow I'm made out to be this monster who did horrible things to you. You've already ruined our relationships with friends and family by telling them all about what I did. You constantly treat me like garbage, and violate my privacy by looking through all my stuff. But I'M the problem?!? Take a look at yourself for once. Maybe when you start looking at yourself you'll find that there was a good reason I did what I did…

Why I'm Different – Sparta, Wisconsin

You've told me I have to go to therapy and sex meetings or we're done. So I've been going. . . I've gone to my fair share of those meetings, even though I really don't know why I'm there. Everyone in those meetings is so messed up, and they've all done way worse things than I'll ever do. It's embarrassing even being associated with those losers.

I know you're upset by all this, but what do you expect from a man?! You knew coming into our relationship that all men cheat. Why would I be an exception? If you could've just accepted that, we wouldn't be where we are today. And don't get me started on our sex life. That evaporated years ago. Suddenly because you found a few emails now *I* am the source of all our marriage problems?! Why don't *you* take some responsibility for what got us here?

How long will this go on? I'll keep going to those stupid meetings and to therapy, but I really hate being controlled by you.

WHO ARE YOU?!?! – Denver, Colorado

WHO ARE YOU? This isn't the woman I married twenty-five years ago. She was so sweet, loving, trusting, fun. She was so carefree. She took everything at face value and always gave me the benefit of the doubt. But now....This same woman is an angry, resentful, depressed...Monster...

I screwed up. I hurt you. But what happened to you??? I want my wife back.

Trying to Explain – Sacramento, California

Hi. I wanted to write you a letter to try and explain. I know you are really mad and really hurt. I never wanted to hurt you, ever. I was sad and lonely. We had moved to Houston where I knew no one. Your job was amazing and you seemed really happy and I was just lost! I don't know if you can empathize and maybe it's not right for me to even try and explain. The kids were so young, I didn't know what I was doing as a mom. I tried but it just wasn't working. And I thought I told you how desperate I was but I am not good at that; I am learning.

Anyway, every day when I would take our oldest to school and then be with the baby, I felt like I was going to die. The baby would go down for a nap and so would I. And then after school, walking to the bus stop, waiting for Sarah to get off the bus and knowing a long afternoon and evening of homework, making dinner and not knowing when you would get home and what your mood would be…I was dying.

I thought I was making a friend with Steve. I was a stay-at-home mom, he was a stay-at-home dad. I'm sorry. And you are right. He isn't the first. I'll tell you as much or as little as you want to hear. I'm sorry.

Vulnerability – Salt Lake City, Utah

You and I have been in sex counseling for a few months now. Everyone keeps talking about "intimacy" and "vulnerability" – I can't tell you how many times those words have come up. I nod my head but I have no idea what those words mean. I know what they mean, but not what they MEAN. You know? Dad taught me to use my fists, to protect myself and fight back. I'm so glad he taught me to stop being such a pussy. He saved my life. I don't know where I'd be without him. Now I hear you and our counselor telling me to "open my heart," be "vulnerable" and talk about my feelings. Well, every bone in my body fights against doing that. It goes against everything I was taught growing up. I don't mean to be stubborn. I hate what I did to you, and I want to do anything to make it better. But I just can't see how being weak makes us stronger.

Pleasing You – Jackson, Mississippi

I just want to get this right! I'm trying so hard now to make sure I have the best therapist and the most recovered sponsor; that I'm going to the correct meetings. And you don't think my therapist is skilled enough, you say you don't like it if there are any women at my meetings. You questioned my choice of a sponsor because he is divorced. So I'm going to change therapists, again. And I'm going to try and find men only meetings. Maybe there's a sponsor who is happily married through all of this. Hell, I don't know.

Is there anything I can do right? And is there anything I can do so you don't leave me?

Staggered Disclosures – Louisville, Kentucky

I want to protect you. You may not see that, and I can see that my behaviors certainly haven't shown that, but I hate seeing you in pain. I suppose that sounds pretty ironic, now that I see you're in the greatest pain that I've ever seen you in . . . But I do want to protect you.

Just the other day you asked me another question about my sexual acting out. Honestly, I thought we were done with the questions, but I answered you regardless. Well, I answered SOME of what you asked. I mean, if I were to tell you the WHOLE truth I just don't think you could take it. So I left out a detail or two.

Again, I want to protect you. How much is it really helpful for you to know, anyway? Does it help for you to know every single detail of my sexual history? Isn't it enough to tell you that it's bad? Why do you need to keep rubbing my nose in it? Sometimes I feel as though you bring these things up on purpose when things are going well only to undermine all the progress we have been making.

I have been going to meetings, starting therapy, and have been sober for 30 days. Why can't we just leave the past in the past? Let's move on and get past this. I won't do it again. Haven't these last 30 days shown you anything?

<u>Why I'm a Sex Addict</u> – Cheyenne, Wyoming

You ask me often about why I chose to act out sexually. Why sex and not something like alcohol? And better yet, why couldn't I simply behave like a "normal" person? How did I even become a sex addict in the first place? I can't tell you how many times I've asked myself the same question! And I don't say that as a cop-out. I really mean that. I'm trying to understand myself how I got to where I am. I'm trying really hard to get to the bottom of this. The answer for now is I just don't know.

It's Not My Fault – Greenville, South
Carolina

I know you think what I'm doing is
wrong. But it's really not my
fault. First, every guy watches
porn. It's just what we do. I watch
porn, my dad watched and probably
still does. Hell, I bet my granddad
even looked at porno magazines!
So, it's not as bad as you make it
out to be.

And, you know how much I like
sex. I like it a lot. And sometimes
you're too tired, or you're mad at
me, whatever. So it's really not my
fault that sometimes I go and, you
know, party it up a bit. I mean,
what's a man to do?

What else do you want from me? – Ames,
Iowa

It's been more than a month now – our
whole life has exploded, and I've changed
everything. I'm going to SAA meetings,
I'm in therapy now, you kicked me out of
the house, I'm doing everything you're
asking me to do. Yet it's still not enough for
you. Nothing I do is good enough for
you. You keep criticizing me. You're
always so angry. What else do you want
from me?!

I've already said "I'm sorry" hundreds of
times, yet you keep replaying the past. I'm
working really hard at moving forward in
our life, but you keep bringing us back to the
past. If I've told you once I've told you a
hundred times – I can't change the
past. When are you going to let it go so that
we can move on?!?

Fix Me First – San Francisco, California

I know you want to go to couple's counseling, but everyone is saying I need to get better first. So I think it is best if you go do your counseling and groups and meetings, and I do mine. That way we will both be better and THEN we can work on the relationship. Don't you think that makes the most sense?

You Did What? – Boulder, Colorado

I cannot believe you went and told my family about me, well really about us. I still believe there's an us! I still want us to be together. How could you have done this?!

So I need to understand, you sent everyone a letter telling them I am a sex addict, that I hired prostitutes and went to strip clubs and had an affair. Tell me how that helped anything. My sister is an absolute wreck, my brother doesn't believe a word of it. Who else have you told without us talking about this first? I thought we would agree to wait and let me tell people when the time was right? Oh my God.

This is going to affect you too. If we stay together, how are we going to have another Christmas with your family, or with my family? I can't believe you did this. I know you're angry with me and you think I have been stalling telling everyone, and I wanted to do this when I was ready. Couldn't you just have waited? I guess that is asking a lot. It just feels like a bigger mess that didn't have to happen.

Empathy...? – Fargo, North Dakota

People keep telling me I need to have empathy. Empathy this. Empathy that. What does that even mean? My therapist tells me to "put myself in your shoes." I want to know what that means, but he might as well be speaking Greek. And it really DOES feel like I'm learning a new language, but it's a language I suck at. I'm trying to learn empathy, yet each time I try thinking about you I end up still thinking about myself. My brain hurts just trying. What's wrong with me?!

Unhinged – Sandy, Utah

So I've been diagnosed now with ADD, PTSD and depression, which may be bi-polar disorder. I feel unhinged. Ironically in my addiction – I felt some form of control. Now I'm just one big mess. Will I be on medications for the rest of my life? Will you stand by me as I battle all of this even though I have hurt you so much? Do I have any right to ask you not to leave? Please don't leave. Please...

I'm Sorry – Las Vegas, Nevada

I'm Sorry. I'm Sorry. I'm Sorry. I'm Sorry. I'm Sorry. I'm Sorry. I'm Sorry. I'M SORRY. I'm sorry…. *I'm sorry.* ***I'M SORRY!*** I'm sorry. i'm sorry. I'm sorry. I'm sorry. I'm sorry. I'm sorry. I'm sorry! I'm sorry……………….. I'm sorry. I'm S O R R Y. **I'm S…O…R…R…Y… I'M** *I'm Sorry.* I'm sorry. I'm sorry……..

60

<u>Unraveling Questions:</u>

For Addicts:

- *What feelings or reactions did you have when reading these letters?*
- *Which letters did you relate most to? Which did you not relate to?*
- *What is missing from each of these letters?*
- *How would you re-write one or any of these letters? We encourage you to get help from a sponsor, trusted friend, or therapist before sharing with your partner.*
- *After answering these questions, please re-read the letters. Read them with an open mind, looking for areas of commonality with your own story. Write down any new insights you take away after re-reading through the letters.*
- *Keep reading! You're on the journey.*

For Partners:

- *Were you able to distinguish the problems with the addict's delivery in these letters?*
- *What is the problem with each letter?*
- *How much anger, fear, sadness, or hope does each letter create for you?*
- *Which letters mimic what the sex addict in your life has said?*

- *What would be good responses for you to these letters?*
- *Which letters and insights would you feel okay sharing with someone you trust?*

PART THREE: PUTTING THINGS TOGETHER

There are so many questions that the addict has and that the partner is asking. The sex addict wonders how he got here, why he does these behaviors and is shocked at the effect this has had on his partner. Most partners want to know everything that happened; what, where, how, when, and with whom. We need to take into consideration that the world she knew and trusted no longer exists. Unfortunately the addiction has polluted every facet of the relationship. She wants "the whole truth." He wants more than ever to console her and make things right.

Disclosure is where the addict tells what he has done. (SEE APPENDIX 3) Unfortunately, this often happens without any guidance. Because he is scrambling to save his marriage or relationship he makes a mess of the information, either giving too little or too much of the right or wrong details. This causes further harm. We encourage working with a skilled sex addiction specialist who can expertly guide this process. Done well, the foundation of trust can start to be rebuilt; done poorly we slide further into more insanity and chaos.

There are many issues that come up at this time, including grief, withdrawal, reactive behaviors by the partner, poor coping skills of the addict, better interpersonal attempts by the addict that the partner can't accept because of her trauma. With hard work, the addict does start thinking and behaving differently. This, thankfully, does get acknowledged by therapists and peers. The pat on the back or sweet hug from his wife, however, rarely is present at this point. We need to pay special attention to fully understand thoughts and feelings as we cultivate a greater understanding of what our faulty way of "being close" was, and embrace a different way of being trustworthy so that our partners can feel safe and lower their defenses.

In New Rules of Marriage *(2008, p 79),* Terrence Real *writes that with conflict in relationship we cannot "fight, flee or fix." We believe these are trauma responses, including the desire to fix things. When we feel our lives are out of control, we are anxious or panicky. For many people there is a constant low level of anxiety that they are rarely aware of. This drives controlling behavior. Considering the context, it is a reasonable response. Living with the knowledge that sex addiction is present in the relationship creates shock, confusion, chaos and instability – all things contrary to feeling safe and secure.*

When we are in trouble, the assumption is that we ask for help. What we see consistently is that the addict's treatment is given priority and the partner puts herself last, repeating a long-lived dynamic of putting others first.

With trust shattered, the partner's thinking can become deprivational, meaning she is in a survival mode with threats appearing everywhere. In this mind state there can be internal and external pressure to not seek out the most comprehensive treatment for the family system. There are many 12-step programs that are helpful in arresting the addiction and keeping acting out behaviors in check. We now know this is a brain disease that needs to be treated by professionals, so it is important to take time to research counselors, doctors, spiritual leaders and treatment programs to make sure that they truly understand and are qualified to treat this insidious and debilitating disease.

Empirical evidence indicates that sex addiction is rooted in traumatic events from childhood and adolescence. We also realize that the effects of being in a relationship with someone sexually acting out can cause complex post-traumatic stress disorder (PTSD). What current scientific research tells us about how the brain works leads us to recommend specific trauma protocols to move and reconstruct stuck thoughts and beliefs. Talk therapy raises much needed awareness, but does not change the repetitive outdated coping skills that lead to poor thoughts and decisions.

In Facing the Shadow (2006, 2nd Ed., pp. 302-303; Reprinted with Permission by Gentle Path Press) *Patrick Carnes provides a general profile of those who have succeeded in recovery:*

- *They had a primary therapist*
- *They were in a therapy group*
- *They went regularly to Twelve Step meetings*
- *If other addictions were present, they were addressed as well.*
- *They worked to find clarity and resolution in their family-of-origin and childhood issues.*
- *Their families were involved early in therapy.*
- *If they were in a primary relationship, the couple went to a Twelve Step couples' group such as Recovering Couples Anonymous.*
- *They developed a spiritual life.*

- *They actively worked to maintain regular exercise and good nutrition.*

All of these components, including actively working toward the restoration of self and relationships are vital for healing the wounds caused by and leading to sex addiction.

For partners...*This is a critical phase for your addicted partner. They are beginning to work a program of recovery, and most likely committed to healing their relationship. This phase is a difficult one for both of you, though, as it will involve some very difficult and painful components: disclosure of hidden secrets, grief, potentially trauma work, clearing up the wreckage of what sex addiction caused, understanding the full relational violation of the addiction, etc. Continue to take good care of yourself in a healthy way as your partner does this work. Don't tolerate abuse if it's in your relationship, but do provide support and patience if possible.*

For addicts... *This is a critical phase. You've been coming out of denial and now you can see the painful landscape ahead of you. Don't turn back. Don't run away. And don't turn on your partner. She's been here with you when - let's face it - you may very well have NOT stood by her side. Keep journeying through and doing the tough work of sharing truth, building accountability, and healing from whatever wounds led you to act out sexually in the first place.*

Disclosure – San Bernardino, California

So here I am writing my "full disclosure," but I had to take a break from that to share this letter. If I'm honest I have to say I don't know what the hell I'm doing. Yet my therapist keeps telling me that you need to hear everything so we can move forward.

How can we possibly move forward when you hear this disclosure? When you hear what I've done, I can't understand why you'd want to stay with me. I've done a lot of s____. I've hurt you. When I write this stuff out I'm shocked by what I see on paper. I wouldn't stay with me if I saw all this stuff, so why would you? How is this helpful??

I love you. I'd do anything to keep you from leaving me. I hate that I hurt you. But I don't know how hearing any of this would help you.

I had to write this to you. Who knows? Maybe this is my last letter to you. I'll keep writing this disclosure to you. Maybe someday you'll see that none of this was about you. But it doesn't look good. Yeah, I'm scared. I'm *scared*! Why would you stay when you hear this? All I can hope for is that you're a better person than me.

That's all I have to say. This disclosure process seems crazy, but I'll do it. I'm backed into a corner so what else can I do? I just hope you know that I didn't push for this and I DO love you. I know it doesn't look like it, but I DO.

I Wanted To Tell – Newark, Delaware

Oh baby there were so many times I
wanted to tell you. Honey it just
rips my heart apart that I lied and
cheated on you. That time you
almost caught me but I told you I
had to be at a meeting in Atlanta,
when I really hopped a plane to
Chicago instead. You called that
evening and I was a wreck. You
were so sweet and told me to go to
bed and have a good rest. Oh if I
had only been able to do that.

I am so sorry. I want to tell you
everything now. This disclosure
thing the therapists are talking
about. I think it will be a good thing
for us both. That way you'll know
all of it all at one time. I know I
have been telling you bits and pieces
and that just isn't right. You need
to know. I know you need to know
but damn if I ain't scared you'll
leave me.

You Scare Me – Detroit, Michigan

I haven't wanted to tell you this. I know how angry you are that I went outside our marriage. What I want to say is that I love you. And I feel intimidated by you. You're smart and successful with your work. You seem able to handle everything. You're attractive and competent.

There are some days I feel I do not measure up.

There are times I feel no matter what I do I am a failure.

I can't possibly make as much money as you, provide for our family as you do, be as good a parent, or have friendships and relationships as deep as yours.

I don't know why you are with me. I feel so much less than you.

I'm not saying this for sympathy or to be convincing. I have to work on my own self-esteem. In the meantime I now know I have put you down in order to feel better about myself. This was and is wrong.

Just Leave Me Already – Chicago, Illinois

I don't know why we keep spinning on this merry-go-round. Both of us are miserable. I obviously can't make you happy, and I just don't know how much more of this I can take. I'm doing everything I possibly can to make it up to you, but it never seems to be enough for you. So why don't we just kill this mercifully?

I feel like you need me to be the bad guy – to leave you and show yet one more way how much of an asshole I am. Well, guess what? I AM an asshole. Who could do what I've done and not be an asshole???

So let's stop this charade. Let's be honest and admit that the damage has been done. I've hurt you beyond repair. I just don't think I can leave you, so let's cut our losses and end this thing…

I Can't Stand It – Birmingham, Alabama

I know you don't want to hear this and you're driving me crazy. I've been sober now for six months. And it has been really hard. You don't want to hear that because of how I hurt you. I'm doing everything!

I need you to leave me alone. Your constant badgering and attacking, I can't stand it anymore. I have to get out of here. I don't know what to say because it's all wrong; I'm too loud or too quiet. I don't come home with the right groceries, or I come home with the right ones but I spent too much. I get what I did was wrong. And I want this to work. And I can't be the only one who has to go to therapy and meetings and say I'm sorry all the time – can I?

I have no idea how we are going to get through this.

I can't do this alone.

You need to get help too.

Surrender – Buffalo, New York

I give up. I've been fighting for so long. And I
don't even know what the battle is about. Please
help me God. I don't know what to do. I feel that
everything I do is wrong and there is no way out. I
don't know how I got here. I feel like a failure. I
feel hopeless. There's a part of me that wants to
die. Still, though, I don't act out. It must be you
that is there somehow keeping me sober. Tonight,
in the middle of the night, I feel my pain. Everyone
else is asleep and I am alone with my thoughts and
feelings. I screwed up. As hard as I try, I am
imperfect

The moon is full tonight. I pray that tomorrow will
shed more light on how we got into this mess. I
know I did some things today that hurt you and I
was so hurt that I lashed out. I'm so tired. I don't
know if we will get through this one, or if I will
lose you. And I have to give this outcome away. I
give it to the moon, to God, to the quiet of the night
to figure out. I love you.

Enough – Fort Lauderdale, Florida

I'm not that good with words. But I'm
going to try. I get that this has been hard for
you. And I get that it's really, really hard to
get over. But I am tired – no, exhausted -
from constantly being told how rotten I am.

I am in recovery. I get that you are scared to
trust me even after all this time. I get that I
have hurt you in ways I will never
understand.

But I'm not going to be yelled at anymore.

I am not going to let you call me names
anymore.

I'm not going to be berated anymore.

I'm not going to be criticized anymore.

Depressed – Tacoma, Washington

I didn't want to tell you because you have been through enough with my addiction. I finally went to the doctor and told all of how I am feeling. He wants me to go on anti-depressants. I thought once the addiction was in check, once I wasn't acting out that everything would be good and now this. I've heard other people in program talk about their medications and I felt proud that that wasn't me.

I don't know what to do. I feel ashamed. I want to blame it on our relationship or the kids or my job. It doesn't matter. I know I need to do something I just really wasn't expecting this.

Tired – Rego Park, New York

I've not been acting out now for a while. The feeling of anxiety I have sometimes is so strong and intense I want to cry and run and hide and kick and scream and just die! I want you to do something about it. I want you to save me from this. I want you to tell me everything is going to be ok; that we will be ok.

And you just look at me. It used to be your eyes would be angry and flashing, but now they are just dull and dead. I don't know why you can't believe me when I say I am really trying and how hard this is!

My therapist says it is because I've been telling you for years that I will get better, and then I have a set-back. So now you don't believe me anymore. I feel awful. And I feel exhausted.

Everything – Rock Hill, South Carolina

I want you to know you were everything to
me. I loved you from the moment we met –
and I knew I would ultimately betray you and
hurt you. You brought me joy, laughter,
security, love. And you supported me when
no one else would or could. The only reason
I can give why I betrayed you was – I was
scared. I remember we were talking about
having a baby, which was terrifying for
me. How could I have wanted something so
badly, which was you and our relationship,
and yet be so terrified of it at the same
time? I think…I lost everything when you
chose to divorce me. I understand your
choice. And I honor it. I wish I had never
cheated on you. Nothing in my addiction
matched what we had. I wish I never had
hurt you. I wish I did not have this thing- this
disease. We could have had everything.

Devastation – Portland, Oregon

I went to work today to a job I hate. My back
was hurting me, again. Our credit card debt is
creeping up, again. My mother called and
yelled at me for her birthday card being
late. When I came home and the house was a
mess, the kids were crying and you were busy
trying to fix dinner. All I could think about
was to get away. All I could think was how
horrific my life is and how helpless I am to
change anything. So I left. And I acted out.

My mind is not my own at these times. It's as
if some foreign thing or person takes over. It's
so frightening to me, the whole of it. The
unmanageability of my life. I've wondered if
I'm depressed, but I can't go there. I've
wondered if I'm just not meant to be married,
and I can't go there either. I've wondered if I
should just be dead. I don't dare go there.

Help! – Gary, Indiana

We keep screaming at each other. We are both
getting speeding tickets. I try to say I'm sorry and it
doesn't help. When we aren't yelling, then there is
this cold, stony silence that I want to run away
from. Some people are telling me this will never
get better and that I should just leave now. Other
people are saying that this will take a lot of time but
if I just stay sober, figure out how I got this way,
then maybe we can still make our marriage work.

I don't know what to do. I don't know how to help
you and you say the cruelest things. Do you have to
keep talking about what I have done? I know what
I did! I do not have to be reminded of it over and
over again.

I'm sorry. You should be able to tell me your
feelings. You need to get help but I don't think
there is anyone that could understand what has
happened. Do you think you should ask your
doctor for help? Do you think we should go to our
pastor? This is so embarrassing for both of us.

And I know you will get mad at me for saying that
too. Because everything I say is wrong.

Empathy - Atlanta, Georgia

You keep telling me that the one thing you really want from me is to give you empathy – to feel the pain you're going through. You say that you really want me to "get it." I know it's hard to believe, but I REALLY WANT TO GET IT TOO! Yet there's some sort of block in me. For some reason I can feel empathy when I talk to other people. Like when I'm with my group, or making a program call, I feel for what the other guy is going through. Yet for some reason I'm blocked when it comes to you. I hate that about myself. I know the one thing you really want from me is the one thing I seem to be so incapable of providing.

My therapist tells me that learning empathy is like learning a new language. I know when I learned Spanish in school it made my head hurt to try to speak it. I spoke in slow, choppy sentences – it was unnatural. Perhaps it's the same with me and empathy. I'm learning "tools" yet you keep telling me that it's like I'm reading from a book or something –it's forced and wooden. And you're right. For some reason it's a lot easier for me to write this here than to feel empathy and express it to you in the moment. I know I'm getting better at it, but I fear that it's too little too late.

More than Sobriety – Flagstaff, Arizona

I'm thick sometimes. All this time I thought
my whole mission was to stay sober. Seemed
clear. I'm good with clear directions as you
know. Stop doing those
behaviors? Check. Done.

So why didn't our relationship get better when
I stopped those behaviors??? I'm now starting
to realize that there's more to this than staying
sober. I can see that our marriage was torn to
shreds by my behaviors. It looks like trust is
going to take some time to rebuild.

So I'm glad I'm sober, but I'm starting to think
that was the easy part. Now we have the
tough work of rebuilding a marriage that I
destroyed. That is, if you can stick with me to
fix this…

I Know You Are Angry – Colorado
Springs, Colorado

You have every right to be. And I
will be here for you no matter what.
I'm here for you. I love you.

You are the one and only one for
me. I am not leaving.

Holding a Secret – Stowe, Vermont

I hear people saying, "You're only as sick as your secrets." I'm not really sure what that means. I feel better when I talk at my meetings, so that makes sense. I'm starting to share more about my past with people. It feels good. But what about this secret: I had a slip the other day. Do you really want to know that? I also hear people say for me to share my secrets except when it would harm others. It'd hurt you too much if I were to share about my slip. That would set us so far back, when we've been doing so well. So I guess it's best for me to not share it with you. It would hurt you too much. I really think it's in your best interest to hold this one in, but I'm still confused about this "rigorous honesty" thing. What does that even mean, and how does it help you to know everything?!

Putting Things Together Questions

For Addicts:

- *Choose 1-2 letters that best identify where you are or were in your recovery process. Why did you choose these letters?*
- *How did you feel reading these letters? Were there ones that were particularly difficult to read? Why?*
- *Were there any letters that were confusing to you? Can you share these with a trusted person (group members, therapist, sponsor, safe family member, etc.)?*
- *Recovery from sex addiction (or any addiction) is a process of grieving. How do you see your grief process unfolding when you read these letters? See appendix 4 for grieving explanation and resources.*
- *After answering these questions, please re-read the letters. Read them with an open mind, looking for areas of commonality with your own story. Write down any new insights you take away after re-reading through the letters and what action steps you are going to take.*

For Partners:

- *What did you experience when reading through these letters?*

- *Can you distinguish between the positive and negative of each letter?*
- *Which letters resonate with you the most? Why?*
- *What body sensations do you notice as you read each letter?*
- *How pulled in or isolated are you feeling right now if you have identified that you are in this stage?*
- *(We mentioned disclosure in this section. Please go to appendix 3 for more information if you would like to go through this process).*

Part Four:

Making Decisions

This next phase of the journey for the individual recovering from sex addiction involves just that – recovery. After the chaos begins to settle and the situation starts to stabilize, the addict must continue to do the work of restoration, for himself, for his relationship, and for all of the other individuals whom he has impacted through his actions while in his addiction and even for some of his actions before he really "got" recovery.

By this point, he has recognized that if he is truly going to heal, it's going to take more than appeasing his partner. He is going to have to do the difficult work of recovery. He will need to continue working a program, which may involve therapy, 12-step meetings, answering to a sponsor, working the steps, building a new healthy community and developing new ways to relate to others. He will also have to travel inward to discover what underlying wounds, trauma, or background led him to turn to an addiction rather than towards vulnerability with other human beings. This phase of the journey is a difficult one, but invaluable. It is here where true and lasting change will occur. He can no longer be the same individual as when the discovery of sex addiction blew up his life and his relationships.

It's important at this phase that the addict continue to understand the relational suffering he has caused by his actions, and to work on healing this damage. For if he solely does the work to heal himself without changing underlying patterns of relating to his loved ones, he will most likely find his relationships slipping further away.

Though this phase is a difficult one, like the new shoot of a plant pushing through the soil, an addict in recovery will

91

build a solid foundation for himself and for his relationships to come.

For partners...*At this point in the process, your addicted partner is "getting it." They are in recovery, and have made strides towards healing relationships with you and potentially others in their life (e.g., family, friends, community). At this stage he can really use support to continue the momentum he is building if it is safe enough for you to give it. If it's not safe enough yet, talk to a trusted support person to see if there are any other patterns of relational damage continuing, or if there are other underlying needs that you have.*

For addicts... *You're on the right path! Celebrate these milestones of recovery. You've fought hard for them. Don't take your foot off the gas pedal, even if you feel like you're ready to do so. Often times at this stage you will need to continue addressing any underlying wounds from the family you grew up with, or childhood, as well as to continue healing your relationship(s) with people around you. Continue making your living amends and doing the good work you have started.*

Figuring It Out – Vancouver, Washington

I wanted to write and apologize. I'm
not sure where to start except to say that
none of this was your fault. I blamed
you a lot. I wasn't happy with my job,
or with our life. I didn't like that you
were successful and I was
struggling. That, along with my
parents' plea for me to be happy, led me
to start seeing other men. I can't
imagine what this is like for
you. Because there wasn't just one, but,
as you know, many. For me to say they
didn't mean anything to me probably
isn't helpful although it is true. I hear
you say 'then why did you do it?' The
only answer I have now is that I felt
alone, confused and they were – just
there. I know it doesn't make sense to
you. I'm so sorry.

Almost – Indianapolis, Indiana

Instead of "I can't believe I did that," my life is now filled with "I almost did that, but didn't." I'm really proud of this! I know you hate it when I tell you how I've accomplished another piece with my addiction. But for me, this is monumental. And everyone else thinks so, my sponsor, program friends, even my family is now hopeful!

I can't believe the difference. It is like backing up from a ledge that I was on. It feels empowering and exciting. It feels like finally I can say "no." I can't expect you to understand. You don't think like I do. That's hard sometimes because there is this piece of me you will never get, and I have to remember that there are many pieces to you that I will never get, especially the pain I have caused.

For today, almost was a huge accomplishment.

I'm Delusional – Omaha, Nebraska

I can't explain what is happening to me but I am
going to try. I've stopped the big acting-out pieces. I
am not going to massage parlors or seeing prostitutes.
And you and I realize this was a really big piece of my
addiction. I felt happy about this and proud. You
weren't as enthused because of the hurt that caused
but I still knew this was really big for me.

Then I was in one of my meetings and a guy started
talking about how after he stopped his "big"
behaviors he had to look at all his behaviors including
looking at porn, flirting with women, complimenting
waitresses and spending too much time on Facebook.
I am being vulnerable and honest saying I was
shocked and scared and angry I think all at the same
time.

Why? Because I thought flirting was part of my
personality and harmless. Because I realize I've been
thinking about scenes from movies we have watched
and playing them over in my head – too much. Now
I'm being told I have to change EVERYTHING.
The way I act, the way I think, the way I feel. I can't
believe how hard this is. And how I somehow
thought I had this under control, had it down.
Sometimes I am such an idiot.

You Were Right – Providence, Rhode Island

I don't want to admit this. As I'm going to 12-step meeting and talking to my sponsor I keep talking about different friends and people from work. My sponsor, he's great, quietly asks me questions like, 'how much do you think this person cares about your recovery?' and 'Sounds like that friend doesn't want to hang out unless there's drinking involved.' Really old relationships that I thought were the best, I'm now starting to question.

When you and I, together, decided I should stop drinking since that was part of my acting-out pattern, I didn't think it would matter. My friends were my friends. But it is dawning on me that the alcohol and checking out women was the core of our connection. That is sad. I still don't want to believe that's all there is! And when I suggest we meet for coffee during the day, or a different restaurant than our usual, Mike, Sam, they don't want to go. And they make all kinds of excuses. What's really starting to bug me is, they blame you. They can't hear this is my choice.

I have to wonder who my true friends are. Who can be with me as I change my life? I feel so much loss and pain as I see who is there for me; for us, and who were arms of my addiction, and that I was encouraging them as well without knowing it or willing to admit it.

You were right. I just couldn't believe you.

Masculinity – St. Paul, Minnesota

I learned how to be a man from seeing
other men in my life. Not what they said,
but what they did. One common
denominator in all of those men I saw on
TV, the way my step-father treated my
mom, and in the friends I had growing up,
was their desire to have women fall for
them. Landing the hot girlfriend or having
a woman fall hopelessly in love was
something that proved how much of a
man we were; how much of a man I
was. And what better way to prove that
than having sex? If women wanted me, I
must really be a man.

When I met you it was amazing – we had a
relationship unlike anything I've ever
experienced. I felt loved,
desired. Complete. You were and always
have been incredible. Yet over time, the
complexities of work, family, bills, friends,
routine, obligations, left sex much lower
on the list of important components of our
relationship. On one level I understood
that, and on another it really rocked
me. What does it say about me as a man
if I'm not having sex? Am I weak? Have I
lost it? How do I really get affirmed by
others around me?

97

I was never aware of these questions, of course, until much later. But what I do recognize now is that I had to come to terms with what it means to be a man. That masculinity is more than a rugged stoic existence. I am slowly learning that my true masculinity also involves intimacy, vulnerability, tenderness, openness, transparency, compassion, empathy, and all of those other attributes I grew up thinking were only for women. I have a lot of work to do to transform my distorted masculinity, but I am at least starting to get how much more of a man I can be if I continue to allow my sensitivity to flourish.

Why I'm a Sex Addict 2 – Toledo, Ohio

Why am I a sex addict? I'm realizing that as long as I can remember I've been this way. I wasn't "born" this way, or anything, yet ever since I masturbated for the first time, I found that sex makes me feel better. I would love to blame my sex addiction on my family – that the abuse I suffered made me this way. And there is some truth to that. I wouldn't have become sexually active so early had I not been abused. Yet there's more to the story. At a young age, I learned that my sexuality was a comfort to me. When people abandoned, abused or neglected me, my genitals were always there. When I learned that I had to fend for myself and couldn't depend on others, I found that I could depend on masturbation, pornography, and/or sexual contact with others. Though it wasn't quite what I was truly hungering for, I really didn't know any better. And as sad as it is, until you, my relationship with my sexuality has been perhaps the most consistent relationship I have had in my life.

Of course, what started as comfort and even protection didn't end up that way. Exploration turned into conquest, and self-soothing turned into shameful isolation. And all the while I functioned "normally." On the outside, I was charming and successful. On the inside, I hated myself and felt completely dead. What was my secret was going to stay my secret. At least until you discovered it. I could write pages and pages about why I became a sex addict, but all I can say is that it started as a way to protect myself from others and even myself. What it became was a monster wreaking havoc on myself and those I care the most about.

Lying – Little Rock, Arkansas

I lied. I've been lying probably all my life. It started when I was young to get out of trouble or to avoid some sort of conflict; that's what my therapist says anyway. What I'm realizing is that I don't even know when I'm lying. Isn't that crazy? I know it's not funny to you; I didn't mean it that way. I'm just saying that this is such a huge realization for me. It's like I'm learning a whole new way of thinking and behaving.

I need you to know I am trying. And I'm learning what lying really means. I'm learning that even not telling you the whole truth is lying. It's risky for me to be totally honest. I'm scared. I'm scared you are going to get mad. I'm afraid you'll tell me I'm still doing everything wrong.

They Are Nothing to Me – Memphis, Tennessee

I am going to try and explain this and I'm not sure I will get it right, I want to try. My acting out had nothing to do with you.

Let me say that again, you are not, nor were you ever, the cause of my addiction.

I hear you wanting to know about them and what we did. A lot of it I don't remember and I know you don't believe me. I'm learning that I wasn't in my right mind when I, as you put it, "had sex with those whores."

I'm getting clearer. I thought they were my friends. They weren't.

I thought I needed them. I don't.

I know in the past I blamed you for why I went to them. That was so wrong. I couldn't answer why I did what I did, so instead I said it was your fault. I was being a coward and you don't now and didn't ever deserve being treated that way.

I'm seeing now that I broke your heart.

I see how I have hurt you. And your pain breaks *my* heart.

Will it happen again? – New Orleans, Louisiana

You ask me if I will ever again do what I did.

If I had ever known what would happen, I would
never have picked up one of those magazines. That
was a long time ago, but I still remember. I didn't
think anything of it back then. We were just
kids. And my dad just laughed when he found us. I
wish he had done something different, but he didn't.

My main goal is to beat this addiction. I don't know
if I can, but I sure want to try. I've hurt you and at
first it looked like I didn't hurt anyone, but now I
know I did. There were great consequences to my
behavior that just now I am able to see. I didn't see it
then, and I sure do now more than I would have ever
imagined.

I have learned that my actions caused consequences
and harm, harm that you think you can never
repair. I have to acknowledge all of these things. I
need to take responsibility.
You ask if I'll ever do those things again, ever hurt
you like I did. I sure hope not and I'm doing
everything I can think of to not repeat those
things. I've gone through too much pain to take that
great a risk ever again.

Old-Timer - Reno, Nevada

So as of today I now have four years of abstinence from my inner circle behaviors. By this point I know well enough that this is a bittersweet milestone for you. I've learned a lot along the way – man, how naive I was to think after one year that you'd be jumping up and down, rejoicing for my "time." That was a huge blow to my ego that day when instead of exuberance you expressed pain.

But I get it. You didn't sign up for a relationship of acting out, but a relationship of honesty, trust, and faithfulness. And sadly I didn't give you that relationship for much of our time together. I'm giving it to you now, for whatever its worth. My living amends is to continue doing the work, to continue going to meetings and bettering myself, to heal the damage I have caused in our relationship. Some days are better than others, but day after day I am working towards that goal.

They call me an "old timer" in meetings now. Seems strange, and it feels like just yesterday that I started going to meetings. I suppose I'm an old-timer because I've been around for a little while and have been able to maintain my sobriety. All I know is that the more I learn the more I realize I have to do. I want you to know that I am committed to keep walking this path. I am committed to you, and to wake up each and every day to take further steps towards my own healing and towards our healing. I love you more than you can ever know.

Love – Houston, Texas

You have asked me what love means to
me. I have always loved you. I know
you don't believe me but it is
true. However that does not answer
your question. Love to me is being
honest, sharing a life together, and
being able to be there for each other. I
have let you down in the worst way. I
want to love you more and better than I
ever have before. I will do anything to
learn how to do that.

I love you.

<u>Telling the Kids</u> – Hartford, Connecticut

At the beginning of all of this I got so mad because you told your friends about my sex addiction. I know now that I only thought of myself. Too often I still only think of myself. But I'm so glad that you told them – you needed their support to help you weather the storm of what I put you through.

I'm ashamed to say it, but part of me wishes you would've told the kids then, too. Yes, it would've been terrible, but it would've saved me the agony of what I'm about to do. I know it's time to share with them what happened. And I know I need to be the one to tell them about it. You've taken the fall so many times for me since you found out about my behaviors. It's time they knew what has been going on. But it's so hard. Not only have I created such pain in you, now I am putting them in the same place. If they were younger, maybe I could justify not telling them that I broke our vows and hurt you. But they know better. They've seen us and are asking questions. I can't keep this from them any longer. I can't. I won't. Lying isn't an option anymore.

So I'm going to tell them in a way that they can hear it. I owe you that much and I owe them that much. I only hope they can start to forgive me down the road.

Time to Tell the Kids – Tombstone, Arizona

We talked about healin' us first before talkin' to the kids. It's been awhile now and I'm thinkin', and my sponsor's thinkin', I need to make amends or do somethin' with Alex and Sarah. It's somethin' we both have dreaded. And you get triggered all over again when I mention it. Do you think they'll be mad? At me, or you, or both maybe?

Well, I've been doin' some writing and comin' up with words that just don't make sense. What the heck am I supposed to say? Your daddy's been looking at porno since he was your age? Or, gee honey, don't be with a fella like me! So much shame comes up about what I did, all over again.

So, I talked to some people and realized this really is not about me! This is about them and how much do they WANT to know. Now I'm not shirkin' anything here. But what I'm thinkin' is I say somethin' like this:

You know how I've been goin' to all those meetings. And you know your mama and I have been havin' some on and off periods here. I did some things that really hurt your mom and I'm making sure that don't happen again. And I'm thinkin' I may have hurt you, too, with how I wasn't there for you in some ways, no, a lot of ways. And I'm sorry for that, real, real sorry. I'm not askin' for forgiveness. And I am sayin' that if you want to ask me anything at any time, you can.

And then tell 'um that I love 'um.

What do you think about that?

It Takes Two (Take Two) – Tampa, Florida

My sponsor told me not to say anything about this, but how can I NOT? I'm SICK of this. All the responsibility gets put on me. Somehow I'm made out to be this monster who did horrible things to you. You've already ruined our relationships with friends and family by telling them all about what I did. You constantly treat me like garbage, and violate my privacy by looking through all my stuff. But I'M the problem?!? Take a look at yourself for once. Maybe when you start looking at yourself you'll find that there was a good reason I did what I did....

Part of cleaning out the wreckage of my past includes making amends for things I've said and done that have harmed others. To do this step-work, I've been looking through old letters and recovery work. I stumbled across this old letter to you and I'm appalled. Yes, these are my words, but it's hard for me to relate to the man who said them.

God, I'm so sorry. I said and did some awful things to you. Not only did I violate our most basic agreements in the relationship before getting into recovery, I also continued to hurt you once we got into recovery. I can barely remember the man who said those things to you, but I can only imagine how many other horrible things I said and did. In my shame I did what I have always done – put the blame back on you. I was such a hypocrite to tell you to look at yourself when I wouldn't even look at my own actions and inactions.

I'll be working on a more complete amends to you. I no longer avoid the pain I've inflicted on you, but I hope that the man I'm becoming will be living amends to you each and every day.

<u>Staggered Disclosures (2)</u> – Louisville, Kentucky

So, I looked back at what I wrote last year about protecting you by not sharing more information about my sexual acting out. I CAN say that I've come to understand things differently than I did then.

It pains me to say this, but when I look back at how emphatic I was about protecting you, the honest truth is that I wanted to protect ME! I was (and still am) terrified to share all of me with you. In sharing all the horrible things I've done to you, why on earth would you want to stay with me? I convinced myself that I was trying to protect you by not sharing information, when really I was trying to keep you from leaving me.

I often wonder why you stay with me, but I am learning. I am growing. I am working to be a better man than I was. And I've learned over time that it's through openness, honesty, and empathy that I help you heal and help restore your trust. So though it scares me to death, I'm open. You deserve my honesty. It's the least I can give you after all that I've done to you.

Long-term recovery – Lansing, Michigan

There are many who wonder if a sex addict can truly recover. I wanted to write and tell you that this is possible. I have been in recovery now for sixteen years and cannot believe I led the life I did. It is hard for me to remember my very bad behavior, which I now realize was a very poor compensation for a wretched internal life.

Now, please hear, I work at it. Every day I work at it. After sixteen years not in the same way I did when I was new in the program. Now it might be saying a little prayer. Noticing a resentment and cleaning it up. Being aware I have been overdoing it and setting a boundary for better self-care.

Most though, is to never, never, never give up. And to remember there is a way out of the pain that does not involve hurting yourself and others.

Our Anniversary – Austin, Texas

You said the other day that our anniversary means nothing to you. That hurt me. I want to understand that, as you say, nothing is the same. And I want to try and explain my experience, what I believe.

Our wedding day was incredibly important to me. Yes I was scared. Yes I was stressed. And I still remember how beautiful you were in your wedding gown. And how happy I was when our picture was taken. I remember pure joy holding you in my arms as we danced, seeing your new ring sparkle. And feeling my own ring, new and shiny. I had hope. I had dreams. Just like you.

I get that what I did reflects on our marriage. I did not think it would or that it did. It was a separate part of my brain. It was a piece of me that had been with me before I met you, like some t-shirt that is outdated, inappropriate and offensive, but I was too immature to know, and too attached to throw it away.

I want us to have a day that represents our commitment, love and union. I don't care what day it is. I want you to feel secure that that day is new and shiny for you and for us. We will create that new day with new rings, new clothes, a new house if you like! And with new dreams. This is what I want.

<u>Gift-Giving</u> – Silver Spring, Maryland

It's embarrassing to say, but this will come as no surprise to you: I'm a terrible gift-giver. This wasn't always the case. I used to be thoughtful with gifts. When we first got together I was romantic and intentional, pampering you with the gifts I would give. It seemed so much easier back then. I'm not quite sure what changed, but along the way it became harder to give you gifts. It wasn't that I didn't care about you. In fact, I think it was actually the opposite: I cared so much that it scared me. In wanting more than anything for you to appreciate my gifts, I froze. I simply couldn't decide what to get you, so I all too often have chosen to do nothing. Even knowing that what you really wanted from me was the opposite, my paralysis still took over.

So here we are in recovery. I know that I've hurt you beyond words through my lies, secrecy, and betrayal. And now it pains me to know that I continue to hurt you further through my poor gift giving. As if holidays like Mother's Day and our anniversary weren't hard enough already, you now have the added insecurity of not knowing what gifts I'll give (if I'll give them at all). All I can say is that I'm working on it, and that it has nothing to do with you. I do love you more than you can know, and all too often more than I can express. Until my gifts match these words, I will keep working to how to show you just how special you truly are.

<u>Pregnancy</u> – Charleston, South Carolina

This letter is painful to write. And I bet it's also painful to read: we're still healing from the pain of my sexual acting out during our first pregnancy. I feel so ashamed to be writing this, knowing that you were at your most vulnerable during this time. You were so joyful, filled with hope. We were beginning a new life together as we took the leap of faith to bring a new child into the world. I can still remember the glow on your face during that time. Your pregnancy wasn't easy, yet somehow you were never more alive.

That all changed when you discovered my acting out. You went from blissful to devastated in a matter of minutes. What I wouldn't give to take it all back. What I wouldn't give for you to have never discovered what I'd done. Most of all, I wish I had never betrayed you in the first place. Words can't gloss over this pain . . .

You ask me time and time again, how I could be acting out during your pregnancy. We were starting our new life together, and how could I have been with other women? All I can say is that I was scared. It terrified me to bring a new child into the world. I wanted to be the best husband possible. I wanted to be the best father imaginable. But then the abuse of my own parents flooded me. The pressure of being someone they weren't was so unbearable, and all the while I feared I would lose you to our new child. I know it sounds incredibly childish. It WAS incredibly childish. I'm so sorry I betrayed you during this period in our lives. I only hope and pray that I can be the best father from here on out, since I certainly wasn't even close to what you (or our family) needed at that time.

It isn't (and wasn't) Your Fault – Brooklyn, New York

One of the best ways I can make amends to you is to finally take responsibility for my behaviors – to acknowledge the many ways I blamed you for what was ultimately mine to own. Though difficult, I hope this letter becomes one small gesture towards healing the brokenness I have caused in you and in our relationship.

Before I got into recovery I blamed you: making you the problem. I made you think that because you were so devoted to so many different amazing activities: our kids, school, work, activities, friends, your dreams, etc., that the disconnect we experienced in our relationship was your fault. Our lack of a fulfilling sex life (let alone our lack of an intimate emotional life) was clearly your doing, since you had overextended yourself. Or so I made you believe. When the years, the kids, and your health difficulties took their toll on your body, I exploited your insecurities.

To hide my own shame at the sexual behaviors I was involved in without your knowledge I turned my focus from myself and instead made you feel bad about yourself. I don't recall what I was thinking during those times, but I know that I felt so bad about myself that I couldn't have you find out about my shameful secrets. I gaslit you. Those three words are petrifying, but they are the truth. I made you think that YOU were the problem, when

117

all along it was really me.

Even into recovery I continued this same pattern. My original game was up, my secrets were discovered. Yet I continued to push you away all the same. What I now know to be your trauma response of hypervigilance, I then labeled you "crazy" and "controlling." "I'm different after all," I told you. "I now have 90 days of sobriety and I'm not that man anymore. Let the past be the past. Why can't you get over it?"

Little did I know then what I do now: how could you possibly know the new man I was in recovery when you were only finding out who I WAS all along? I continued to push you away, blaming you and manipulating you through exploiting your insecurities. And as only intimate partners can know, I knew your deepest darkest secrets and vulnerabilities. And I exploited them.

I AM a different man now, but I'll let my actions show that to you. I have deeply hurt you, wounding you deeper than perhaps anyone else ever could. I hate that that's the case, but I want to fully acknowledge that. I also want you to know that you are incredible. The strength you have shown: the faith, the ability to find yourself again, and ultimately the ability to trust others again – I'm baffled. You are so incredibly strong and brave. And you were right all along.

I deeply, deeply apologize for how I have hurt you. I hope each effort I make to acknowledge your reality helps to delicately put back a shard of broken glass to put back together your shattered world.

I'm Sorry – Miami, Florida

God, I can't say that enough. I think I will be saying I'm sorry until one of us is dead. I can't, myself, believe what I have done. Now when I look back, my acting out seems like a dream, a horrible nightmare. You ask me repeatedly how I could have done those things. How could I have violated our marriage vows? Didn't I realize what was at risk? The answer is "no." I did not think of anything when I was in the addiction, not you, not the children, not our families, not my reputation, nor yours. My mind went blank; fuzzy; even sort of spacey. I had no control. For you this is unconceivable. Because you are great at handling stress, you always have been. And I have leaned on you to pick up the extra pieces.

Anyway, this time is very confusing for me and I am getting better at realizing my thoughts and patterns and what triggers the addiction for me. I am focused on getting better and not doing anything to hurt you again, ever.

A thousand times, I am sorry.

Depressed (Revisited) – Tacoma, Washington

Depression . . . I know I wrote about this once before. Seems like ages ago now. I also know a little bit more about my depression, and I wanted to share with you what I've been learning. I don't share this to justify my behaviors or anything, since what I did to you was 100% mine to own. But I did want to share more of myself with you as I practice vulnerability.

Looking back on my life, I can see how I have always been depressed. I didn't know it at the time, but getting in fights, withdrawing into my room, escaping into drugs with high school friends, and discovering porn were all ways of masking my depression. For just a few moments I could escape myself, occupying another world where my pain didn't exist.

My therapist keeps talking about my "family of origin" and how my family played into my depression. At first I wanted to defend my family. And unfortunately, you know that I've done that even in our relationship – abandoning you to protect them. Well, the reality is this: they did their best, but they also really didn't do that great of a job with me. Emotionally neglecting me and not protecting me from the sexual abuse I experienced from my uncle were ways they really hurt me. And now that I look back on it, I can see that depression showed up for me pretty early on. And though I didn't know what depression felt like, I did learn about how I could avoid the pain.

I recognize now that in working so hard to avoid pain, I developed an addiction to sex. And I hate to think that my addiction has now caused even more pain to you than I ever could have imagined. I want you to know that part of my living amends to you is to continue healing my past so that I no longer inflict on you further pain from my addiction.

Shame – Baton Rouge, Louisiana

If ever there was a tough topic to write to you about, it's shame. Even saying that word in my mind conjures up this image of a giant black gorilla, reaching out to clasp at my throat. It's a suffocating feeling. How else can I describe it to you but to say that when I feel shame I simply disappear? Don't get me wrong, I'm still there with you when I go into shame. Well, at least I'm partially still there. I hear the words you're saying to me, but somehow they're a hollow and distant metallic echo – like you're talking to me from across a tunnel. I'm a fraction of who I was before I went into shame.

Shame scares me. Admitting that is difficult, but it's true. I am so filled with shame and remorse, and even before realizing that what I was experiencing was shame, I knew it was a monster not to be reckoned with. I never really learned how to deal with shame. Unfortunately, what I did learn was this: acting out sexually helped diminish my shame, at least until it was over and the flood of shame assailed me again. It was an endless cycle that ensnared me.

I want you to know that my shame is mine alone, and not yours to hold for me. I've defended against my shame in many different ways: blaming you, defending myself, shutting down, shutting you down, and getting depressed come to mind as a few of those ways. I'm sorry for how I have taken my shame out on you. Prior to recovery it was simply too overwhelming for me to hold. Yet I recognize now that this shame is mine, and I'm working on it. More

123

than anything I want to be able to hear your pain, hold your anger, and comfort your feelings of betrayal. And I will continue to tear down brick by brick the wall of shame that prevents me from being there for you.

Making Decisions Questions:

For Addicts:

- *What feelings or reactions did you have when reading these letters?*
- *Did you see hope in any of these letters? How does it feel to have hope?*
- *When reading these letters, did you think anything they were saying was weak, a cop out, stupid? Which letters and why?*
- *Were any of these letters difficult to understand? Which ones?*
- *After answering these questions, please re-read the letters. Look for areas in common with your story. Write down any new insights you take away after re-reading through the letters and what actions steps you are going to take.*

For Partners:

- *What feelings or reactions did you have when reading these letters?*
- *Which letters would you most want to hear from your partner? Why?*
- *In what letters did you see hope?*
- *What positive recovery do you see in your partner? What would you still like to see?*
- *In these letters do you hear any vulnerability, honesty, and humility? Where?*

Part Five:
Moving Forward

So far we have covered the beginning stages of this process, which describe the first years of the addict who is ready to commit to recovery and the right people and interventions are put in place. There IS controversy in the therapeutic community about what treatment should look like. Some think the partner and addict should be doing separate work first before engaging in any couples therapy. Recently we have seen the benefit of seeing the couple together, if both are willing, at least one time per month. The authors are strong proponents of group therapy, especially for the addict. What works for the partner is still being explored. At the time of this writing there are support groups in the United States and Europe and some online. The clients we have worked with say, for both the men's and women's groups, that the benefit of attending support groups is finding others who "get it." This is a lonely experience with not many people who understand and are willing and/or able to offer support. With any catastrophe we look to the people we love and care about to be there for us. With sex or porn addiction, support seems to be polarized to either "Leave him/her" or "Well, that's not that big a deal!" Both are unhelpful.

We now realize that the addiction is rooted in traumatic experiences. "Addictions always originate in pain, whether felt openly or hidden in the unconscious....A hurt is at the center of all addictive behaviors," says Gabor Mate. (In the Realm of Hungry Ghosts. 36, 38.) *Many partners, upon hearing this, are unimpressed and feel this is an excuse. What we have come to learn in our practices is that the addict and spouse have very similar wounding at the same developmental stages when they were growing up. The historical similarities are uncanny. A specialized clinician*

129

can sketch out the hurts that are often minimized or overlooked by the client. Getting sent to your room for having done exploratory touching is enough to cause significant shame that can result in hiding any and all sexual behavior from then on. Men being teased about their penises, even if the adult was "just playing" can result in a compulsive desire to be seen, potentially leading to exhibitionism. We are redefining what love and nurturance is and how stress and technology are affecting individuals and families. Needless to say, the addict and the partner will need to address and heal from the current trauma and any similar past trauma. The brain congeals current traumatic events with ones that are similar from in utero onward.

Few couples file for divorce immediately upon hearing of the betrayal. The first thought is to seek out a couples' therapist. More marriage counselors are learning about sex addiction and the training and competency is diverse. We encourage you to seek out a highly trained sex addiction therapist. The authors are both Certified Sex Addiction Therapists (CSAT) trained by International Institute for Trauma and Addiction Specialists (IITAP). This training is rigorous and thorough with demanding continual education requirements to be kept current on the latest research and treatment protocols.

There are many experiences that happen for the couples from discovery onward. Many addicts get frustrated by the partner's anger, depression, regular and repeated questioning and threats of leaving. There are three major questions that the partner is asking under ALL of it. These are: **Do you love me? Do you want to be with me and only me? And, Are you going to leave me?** *If the addict* can remember these pleas are at the core of all the partner's outward unpleasant behavior, healing will happen more quickly. If she has not taken off her engagement and wedding ring, and has not filed for divorce, you are still married.

Talking to family members, especially children, teens and young adults can be difficult and awkward. The family interacts and experiences its members relationally. Anyone who believes the kids are not affected is sadly mistaken. We are constantly picking up on non-verbal communication and at the very least, children will experience the addict as being "absent" during the addiction with the partner overcompensating and stressed. After discovery it is impossible to cover the myriad of emotions that are happening for both adults. We have discovered that even pets are affected by the impact of sex addiction with symptoms such as heart problems, digestive challenges and diagnoses of cancer. The discussion of the addiction needs to be well thought through with awareness and care of what developmental stage the child is in, how much they have been exposed to the addiction, and how ready and willing they are to know what has happened. We often find it helpful for both parents to be present when the addict talks with the kids. We want to take special care to be ready to be appropriately honest and to listen closely to how the children are feeling about what happened, and then how they are experiencing the changes happening in the family.

For partners...At this point, you are in a new phase in your own healing and in the healing of your relationship. You don't see things the way you once did. Though we'd *never wish you to have to walk the road of sexual addiction in your relationship, you have clearly done good work to get here. You've found hope. If you're able, please share this hope with other partners who are in the earlier stages of the process and need to grasp some of what you have.*

For addicts*... You have worked hard to get here – Harder than maybe anyone will ever know. Keep up the good work! Even though working your recovery won't be as "hard" as it once was, don't underestimate the value of what you have. Take what you have and give to others who are struggling to "get it." Share your renewed vision of yourself, your relationship(s) and the world with others still in the dark. Congratulations! All the difficult work you've done is paying off in your life – maybe differently than you expected, but the trust you have is even more deeply satisfying than you ever dreamed possible.*

<u>The Gifts</u> – Palisades, New Jersey

We've been in this for a while now, and with sobriety has come a renewed clarity in my life. I finally get how absent I've been through much of our relationship. I abandoned you not just when I acted out in my addiction, but also through how I withdrew from you emotionally, mentally, and spiritually. I rejected and neglected you.

Though I am by no means perfect right now (you can attest to that!), each day brings a new opportunity for me to continue healing the wreckage of my past. And it's so painful for me to know that much of the wreckage comes from what I caused in our relationship.

I wouldn't wish this addiction or its destructive impact on anyone, yet I do see our "D day" as a gift. I hate that I caused you so much trauma through my addiction, but your discovery began my healing and our restoration. I so wish we could've walked a different path to get to where we are, but I want you to know how dedicated I am to our healing. The gift of this pain is an intimate relationship like we'd never known. I love you so much.

133

What Have I Missed – Washington, DC

I wanted to write to you about something important. It has been brought to the forefront of my awareness that through my addiction, I have been absent, not here, not totally with you. And in that oblivion, I have missed so much.

The relationship we have today is like no other. Certainly it is different from anything I have experienced. The caring, love, connection I feel with you is exquisite! I used to laugh at romantic comedies; I used to make fun of men who cried; I used to berate my male friends for being sentimental or affectionate towards their wives. How stupid and shallow I was.

Our life together means everything to me. I see you more clearly now than I ever have before. I accept you and I am learning to accept myself. The time we have together is fresh, new, and precious. I knew before how much I hated being alone. Now that has changed to I don't like being alone, but I'm okay when I am – and I love being with you.

Finally – Redding, California

We are in such a better place. I do not ever want to go back to our former life. What pain and misery! I am happy that when I say that now, you agree. I am grateful that you have stuck by me. This was not easy for either one of us. I think the worst was seeing your pain and knowing my addiction caused it. I say "my addiction" now instead of "me." And we are both in agreement that my behaviors were not really who I am.

Time has passed and it is hard for me to believe what I did. It seems like a dream - a nightmare, really. I look back and see how my thoughts led me to dark places. I can kind of see how I could justify things and from this place, all of it appears crazy! When I tell my story at meetings, I still realize what I did and that time seems so very far away. I want to say that it didn't happen. I want to say it was not me. But I know it was. I never want to be in that place again. And I want you to know I am doing everything I can to make sure that I do not repeat the past.

The Bigger Picture – Provo, Utah

This thing goes so much further than just me. I realize now that my sexual activities affected way more people than I ever thought possible. First and foremost, my acting out harmed you. It damaged your trust and our relationship, and even how you see yourself and others around you. It hurt our kids. All that we've gone through because of my addiction has taken a toll on our family. They've suffered through my years of being absent when I was acting out and they've suffered now as we've stumbled to right the sinking ship of our marriage. My addiction has affected our relationships with our family and our friends. We've lost friends and family members because of what I did. I also realize now that my sexual acting out reinforces a system that says it's ok for men to cheat on their wives. And unfortunately, I've contributed to a world that has made that okay. And that's the world our son and daughter are stepping into.

This addiction has taken a terrible toll. I understand that now. I only wish I could've seen this then. I'm grateful for the friendships we have gained, for our renewed relationship,

136

and for the man I have become. I am working each and every day to make society a better place for our children and our children's children. I believe we all are capable of changing, and I am infinitely grateful that you have believed enough in my recovery to stay by my side in spite of all I've put you through. You are incredible.

Remember? – Charlotte, North Carolina

I have been thinking about where we were and where we are now. I used to come home from my 12-step meetings and just go to the kitchen and get a snack, while you sat alone, waiting, in the living room. I was sober! I talked with people at the meeting, including my sponsor. So I thought all was good!

Now I realize what it means to connect. I look forward to coming home and sharing with you what our topic was, how I felt about it, and what thoughts and feelings came up for me. This has been such a big change! I didn't realize I was withholding and withdrawing. I guess this is because I was raised to just shut up and be quiet and to stay out of trouble. But in that process I never got heard and that's a big problem. I'm happy that you listen and don't say negative things anymore about my program. Thank you for that. I now know how hard this has been for you with new therapists and new friends, having to figure out who to tell and what to tell over the years. All the money spent on therapy and all the time I have had to spend on reading and writing, talking to other people and you trusting those calls are all about recovery.

Thank you for your patience and support.

I love you so very much.

It Wasn't "Fun" – Beverly Hills, California

I've been thinking a lot these days about
my addiction. After receiving my five-year
chip I thought I should look at who I am
now versus who I was then. I've been
around these rooms long enough to know
that people outside these walls often don't
"get it." Just as I didn't have any idea
what I was doing and why I was doing it,
most people out there – friends, family,
and the media – also don't get what sex
addiction is.

I hear a lot of people saying, "Isn't calling
sex an addiction just a way for a jerk to
get off the hook for his bad behavior?" Or,
"If sex is a good thing, how could it
become addictive?" I'm sure I even said
some of those things in the past as
well. YES there are some guys out there,
and some of them have (briefly) even come
through these rooms who are just
assholes. But they don't last long in
program. They don't do the hard work it
really takes to do recovery – to man up
and heal their relationships, their families,
and their own demons.

I know for me and many others that I've
come to know over the years, that sex
addiction was all about pain. It wasn't
"fun." I hated myself before, during, and

after I would act out. I was trying to
numb the pain of my abusive past. Does
my past justify my behaviors? No, not at
all. I'm responsible for everything I
did. But I do see now that when everyone
I was closest to growing up abandoned
and rejected me, I found that I could feel
just a little better when I had sex. It didn't
solve the bigger issues I needed to deal
with, but I wasn't ready to face that pain.

But here I am. I've done a lot of work, and
I can see why I did what I did. I daily
make amends for my actions and what
they've done to you and others in my
life. And as I work on loving myself more
and more, I have opened up a whole new
world where I can now love you like I was
never able to before.

Making Amends to the Women I Have Harmed –
Tulsa, OK

You have said that you couldn't believe I would
look at porn and go to strip clubs when, one, your
values were so feminist and aligned with women's
rights, and, two, that you believed I had those same
values. I have tried to figure this out for myself.
And in the addiction, which was utterly selfish, I
just didn't care. And that was wrong.

We are no longer together, but I still wanted you to
know I am sending money to Breaking Free, the
Centre to End All Sexual Exploitation, and
Treasures.

I've also started volunteering at the church youth
group and plan on talking to the young men about
pornography. I want to be real with them and not
simply be another adult preaching to them. I don't
know if they will hear me, but I need to try and
explain how devastating this can be.

I'm telling you this not for validation or recognition
but to let you know I want to do the right thing. For
you to realize I was listening to you. And for me to
be in line with my real values, even though I strayed
so far from them.

I want you to know that I appreciate your wisdom,
your honesty, and your healthy attitude.

Recovering my Self-Respect – Ojai, California

It's true – I started recovery for you. I went to meetings, and even went to the therapist you found for me, all the while acting like a spoiled teenager sent to his room. I gave the therapist a hard time and I took it out on you. As if somehow YOU were punishing me for my misbehaviors. I've done a lot of growing up since then.

You need to know that though I'm committed to US, I'm recovering for ME. I don't mean that selfishly or narcissistically. I mean that I'm finally recovering some self-respect. I no longer do those things that hurt you so badly. I try so hard to say what I mean and do what I say. I try to show through my consistent trustworthy actions that you can rely on me. I never take that for granted. But I'm healing for me.

Even as I write this I have a visceral experience of disgust at who I was and what I did. I know I have an "addict" part of me, and I now understand him and why I did what I did. Of course that doesn't justify any of my behaviors. I am still fully responsible for all the actions and the pain that I caused you and our family. But I'm disgusted by how I "coped" with life. I'm not that guy and I respect myself and you too much to ever go back. I will work each and every day in my recovery to be the man that I always wanted to be, the man you always thought you had. I AM that man now. Thanks for standing by me while I became that man.

Humanizing Women – Pittsburgh, Pennsylvania

Over the years in my recovery, I've learned how important it is to "humanize" women (well, everyone really). From my secretary to my acting-out partners, and at times even you, I treated people as though they existed to meet my needs. I realize how much of my life I have spent objectifying others. When people weren't safe growing up, I found ways of manipulating and using them. I carried that pattern into our relationship, and can now see so many times where I did the same thing to you.

I know I still have work to do on this, and will probably be doing it until the day that I die. But I'm committed to this work. I'm committed to you. I'm committed to letting you see just how important you are. You need to know that I've stifled you. I've suppressed you. I've put you down, and in my insecurity to let you shine, I've put out your flame so many times. In my insecurity, your gain was my loss. I mistakenly thought that if you were to realize your full potential that you would have no need for me. I devalued you. I know that now.

In all this work that I've done, I can see my own value. And as I see my own value I'm not threatened by yours. I so want to undo the damage I've done – to continue to build you up. You're beautiful. You're amazing. You're the best decision I've ever made.

I now see you more clearly for who you are. And I want to see others more clearly for who they are. The gift of this recovery to me is seeing you and each human being that I come into contact with as a full human being. I know it will surprise you to hear me say this, but I'm not the center of the universe.

Grateful – Topeka, Kansas

Today I'm grateful. I have a full life. I have true friends who I can laugh with, complain to, have deep conversations about how I feel. I think back to when I was in my addiction. I couldn't talk to anyone, or so I thought. I monitored everything I said feeling out the other person's reaction first. Those days seem pretty far away today.

Today I'm grateful for what I have. My life is fairly simple compared to others. We live in a three bedroom house and I'm happy. My job is good! I'm able to get along with the people I work with. Yes, sometimes I have a hard day. And I realize "Wow! Today was rough!" and I can go for a walk with the dog, look at the moon (it was full tonight by the way, just beautiful), talk with a program person, do some writing and then put the day into perspective. I can see what I can control and what I can't and be okay with it all.

I'm grateful I'm not alone. I know now there are so many people and forces at work that really want me to be safe and taken care of. I realize I don't have to be so much better to be loved. I realize I'm doing the best I can to be compassionate, kind, and loving towards others and most of all to give myself permission to make mistakes…to not always have the answer and sometimes to inconvenience others although I don't mean to. I also realize, and this is huge, that I can't control how other people feel. That, in itself, is a huge relief.

Thank you for staying with me, when you didn't have to. I'm grateful for you having been in my life and still being in my life. You are the most beautiful person I know.

Gratitude - San Francisco, California

I'm grateful that you stayed

I'm grateful you have been such an anchor in our relationship

I'm grateful that despite the damage I caused, you continue to work on healing

I'm grateful for how amazing you are with our kids

I'm grateful for your smile

I'm grateful for your touch

I'm grateful for getting us into recovery

I'm grateful for your perseverance in recovery

I'm grateful you patiently gave me time to restore our relationship

I'm grateful for your trust

I'm grateful I have each and every day to be the partner you deserve

I'm grateful for your friendship

I'm grateful for the years we have left

I'm grateful for your heart

I'm grateful for your faith

I'm grateful for our shared love of travel

I'm grateful for the spark in your eyes
returning

I'm grateful for that you have such great
friends to turn to

I'm grateful for your strength

I'm grateful for our future

I'm grateful that you're the most amazing
person I know

I'm grateful for our morning coffee

I'm grateful for our check-ins

I'm grateful for falling asleep with you

I'm grateful for laughter

I'm grateful for our shared tears

I'm grateful for our intimacy

I'm grateful for your life

The New Me – Montpelier, Vermont

Sometimes I'm just not sure you're ready for the new me. I've been working on my recovery for more than three years now, and I can finally say that I'm proud of who I am and who I am becoming. I know I've still got work to do, but each and every day I am doing that work. I'm committed to my recovery, to healing our relationship and our family. When I'm wrong, I promptly admit it.

Yet I still feel a wall between us. I've hurt you immensely; that I know. We've been to counseling and have been working on our relationship. But sometimes I wonder if what I did to you was just too much. I know more than to say you're not working on "your side of the street" – man did that blow up in my face when I stupidly brought that up early on in our healing. But you haven't been to therapy in years. Our couples counseling fizzled what feels like ages ago. I know in the past I needed to work extra hard to get sober and to heal the damage I did to you. But now I feel like I'm the only one working at this. It may just be my distorted thinking, but when I try to be vulnerable, I only feel distance or anger from you. Maybe the trauma of what I did is just too great . . .

I believe we can get past this, but I need for us to fight together for our relationship.

What Sex Addiction Stole – Tallahassee, Florida

My sex addiction has robbed you of so much. I see how it has made you question yourself and your judgment. I see how it has made you question the way you see your own body. I see you compare yourself with all the other women out there. I see how it shattered your trust in me. I see how it has distanced you from your friends and family. I see how it shattered your faith in God. I see how my addiction has thrown you into a spiral of pain, anger, and depression. I did that.

I can't undo what I've done. I wish I could – I would do anything to know then what I know now. I was so clueless then. I see my distorted thinking and how I would blame, judge, or criticize you. I wish I could have seen the beautiful, smart, talented, creative, amazing woman then that I see now. I could have spared us so much pain.

I know that we're in a different place now. I'm better than ever, and I see us closer than ever before. But I also know that the cracks I laid in the foundation of your view of yourself and the world run deep. My actions have made you think you were defective in some way. But you need to know that this is the lie of sex addiction - it was never YOU who were defective. It was me trying to fill up a defect in MYSELF that was the problem. I strayed from our relationship because of a problem in me, not because of a problem in you. But I'm here now, and I'm here to stay. Until my dying breath I will do everything I can to show you through my actions just how incredible you are.

BEAUTY – Grand Junction, Colorado

When I think of my "pre-recovery" self, I wish I could say that guy was just clueless. I most definitely was clueless, but unfortunately I did so much damage before I really started to "get it." Though I know the man before you now can't undo what I've done in the past, I do hope that the honesty and integrity can provide you a measure of safety for our future.

One thing I've been thinking a lot about lately is beauty. I know that word has carried a lot of weight and pain for you over the years. What I got to thinking about was how much that word has changed for me. I used to view beauty solely as body parts. I missed all that was around me, all that you are, and traded that for something so superficial and fleeting.

You are incredibly beautiful. Yes, we've both weathered some years. But you are more beautiful today than ever before. I see the light in your eyes, still burning bright. I see the depth of your soul – you have such wisdom. I feel your compassion towards our kids and for those who have less than we do. You have such a presence about you that permeates a room. In the past I spent all my time trying to soak up people's affirmation to feel better about myself, and I missed the beautiful person who was right beside me the whole time. I don't know how you've managed to become even more attractive physically in your 60s than you were in your 20s, but here you stand before me. You are such an incredibly beautiful wife, mother, friend, lover and partner on this journey. I'm so grateful that through these trying years the spark in your soul burns brighter than ever. You are so beautiful.

Hope – Albany, New York

How different hope looks for me now than it did after discovery. I used to think (and tell you), "What's done is done. Why can't you just get over this and move on?" I know now that our "moving on" looks so much different than I ever thought.

I now know that hope for us isn't pretending I didn't hurt you in the ways I have through my sexual behaviors. It's also not about trying to put a quick bandage on all of this. No, hope for us has come through me healing from my past, understanding the impact of my addictive behaviors, and helping you heal from what damage these behaviors did to you and to us. This hasn't been easy. We're still working on it. But I also feel a closeness to you that I've never experienced before. Our intimacy was forged through pain, but it is stronger now than ever.

I would give anything to undo the pain that I've caused you through my betrayal. I would never wish that on you again. Unfortunately I can't undo the past, but I can continue to show you consistently trustworthy actions over time and continue to provide you safety in our relationship as we deepen the intimacy in this new relationship we've developed in recovery.

THIS is hope – you're healing, I'm healing, and we as a couple are healing. We have a future in front of us I never dreamed possible.

Confession – Raleigh, North Carolina

I wanted to write to you because I have always wanted to tell you who I am and also who I was afraid of being. For so much of my life I have lived a lie and been impersonating someone else. I've always been afraid that I wasn't good enough. It's a secret fear that I learned to cover as a child and didn't stop until I got into recovery. Recovery, sobriety. I've said these words so often they now seem hollow. Here's the truth. I'm broken. Even though I've been sober for twenty years now, I'm still broken. All the therapy and meetings will never change that. But there is a huge difference now, which is that I now know and accept that I will never be perfect. It was the striving to be perfect and to fit in that led me down this horrific path.

I'm not good at cleaning the house, or the car. I'm anxious when I meet new people. I drive too fast. I am not good at handling conflict, I have to practice what to say to you or the kids when I'm upset. Instead of acting out sexually, I have now had to face overeating, spending money irresponsibly. There is a difference now though. I'm here. I'm with you. I see you. I see what a smart, beautiful, loving person you are. I see how much you give to people unconditionally. I see how hard you work on yourself. And I see how you are taking care of yourself.

I love the time we spend together. I feel comfortable and connected to you. We have weathered what I think is the impossible. And it's the little things like how you run your fingers through your hair when you are thinking. It is the words you use to describe the artwork you love so much. It's the love and affection you show and extend to our dog and seeing the joy he brings to you. I don't know if I can ever light up that wick of happiness for you again, but I hold hope that our love and trust for each other will continue to grow.

Not Asking Forgiveness – New York, New York

It has been a number of years now since we divorced. I can't say whether it was the best thing or not. I know you went through unbearable pain with what I did. I'm sorry. I didn't mean to hurt you.

I have heard you are remarried and I am happy for you. I hope you have learned that men can be trusted and that they can be good. The kids tell me you have moved on and I am glad. I wish that you have a good life. They say it's the best revenge.

This letter is not to ask you to forgive me, because what I did is not forgivable. I only ask that you live a full life; that you know you are loved, even though I could not show you that as much as I would have wished. You are a beautiful, brilliant, capable, talented woman who has much to give to her partner, her family and the world. I wish you all the best.

<u>Moving Forward Questions:</u>

For Addicts:

- *How do these letters inspire and motivate you in your recovery?*
- *How do these letters inspire and motivate you in your relationships?*
- *What fears do you have about being able to get to this place?*
- *Write a letter of your own from this place in recovery. If you are not at this place, imagine yourself writing as if you were. What feelings come up for you?*

For Partners:

- *Knowing now that this type of intimacy is possible, how do you feel?*
- *Which letters would you most like to get from your partner? Why?*
- *How do you express this need to him/her?*
- *Do you believe such recovery is possible?*
- *What letter would you like to write back to your favorite in this section?*

Afterword

We have explored the addictive journey through five main phases: Being in the dark, the relationship(s) and lives of the sex addict unraveling, the addict beginning to put things together, taking steps towards making important decisions, and finally, moving on towards health in relationships, families, overall life, and in communities.

The journey of a sex addict, and likewise the journey of his or her loved one, is difficult. It may feel like walking into a cave where darkness envelops the light. The "hope" shared in meetings, from friends or families, or even by therapists, feels like words spoken in a foreign language, swallowed up in the shattered world that is impacted by the sexually addictive behaviors. Is this the partners' experience?

Our aim in writing this book was to give a full portrayal of sex addiction from a personal raw perspective. Of course, in order to convey an accurate picture of the mindset of a sex addict, we cannot shy away from the dark side. The pain that partners, families, and addicts experience is very real, and truly devastating. But that's not where the story ends. We wanted to provide the entire experience of the journey and illustrate the developmental stages in sobriety and recovery. We have worked with many men and women on that journey. The dark days CAN and DO lead to the light. The light we see comes in the beauty of intimacy, having joined together with your partner through perhaps the worst days of your lives. This intimacy is forged in truth, honesty, empathy, and an openness to the other. This illumination also reveals itself in a renewed understanding of self. The work done to create this new self, expands to all areas of life – family, relationships, work, and the greater community. We've seen the result of dedicated work bring relationships even closer together – severed bonds built stronger than ever imaged. As clinicians we hold hope with all our clients because we witness change every day.

We hope this book has helped you to see into the mind of a sex addict. If you are someone struggling, we encourage you to get help immediately, so that you can avoid the damage of what discovery, or repeated discoveries, can do to you and to those who love you. If you are a partner or family member of someone who is addicted to sex, we hope this book gives more of a road map for what you can expect at each phase of the journey. Most of all, we want you to know that you're not alone. There are many brave men and women around you who are doing the hard but rewarding work of recovery.

Lastly, please know there are many roads for help. Whether you are an addict, male or female, or a partner, there are therapists, groups, programs, websites, webinars, books, and articles for you. More resources become available every day as professionals and communities realize the support that is needed. Please access our resource list and reach out. And never, never, never give up.

Appendix 1

Healthy Self-Care Activities

My Ways of Relating to Others in a Healthy Way:
(What ways do you turn to others to build up a support
network rather than isolating? Example: Going to
fellowship after meetings, calling a supportive trustworthy
friend, working with a sponsor, being vulnerable with your
partner, asking for help, etc.)

_____

_____

_____

_____

My Therapeutic and Recovery-Based Items:
(What supports do you have through recovery and/or
therapy? Example: Going to therapy, going to meetings,
working the steps with a sponsor, sponsoring others, etc.)

_____

_____

_____

_____

My Ways of Nurturing My Physical Health:
(What ways do you take care of your body in a healthy
way? Example: Getting regular exercise, eating balanced
meals, getting adequate sleep, etc.)

_____

_____

_____

_____

_____

My ways of Managing Stress and Emotions:
(How do you manage overwhelming emotions, relational
stressors, or other vulnerable states? Example: Meditating,
journaling, progressive muscle relaxation, going for a walk,
creating, allowing yourself to cry, taking deep breaths,
grounding yourself by putting your feet on the floor and
hands on your seat, etc.)

_____

_____

_____

_____

_____

My Estimable Acts, Fun, and Passion:
(What ways do you develop and engage in hobbies, foster healthy passion, and give back to others? Example: Doing service projects, developing new hobbies, spending time with family and loved ones, etc.)

_____

_____

_____

_____

_____

My Spiritual Development / Fulfillment:
(What ways do you nurture your faith/spirituality and build deeper meaning in your life? Example: Prayer, meditation, engaging your religious community, retreats, finding purposeful fulfillment, etc.)

_____

_____

_____

_____

_____

Affirmations:

(Affirmations are an important tool. They are powerful messages that confirm you are worthwhile and deserving; that who you are today is okay and enough. Affirmations serve to replace old messages and judgments that feed a destructive mindset. What affirmations can you make about yourself today? Example : "I am enough," "I am worthy," "I am lovable," "I can get through this," "I belong," "I deserve to be loved," "I am okay, just as I am," "I am valuable," "I am aware of the consequences of my actions," "I am whole," "I matter," etc.)

_____

_____

_____

_____

_____

Appendix 2

Options for Spouses and Addicts

Stretching

Running or walking as if you were being chased–engaging flight response

Warm water – over hands/arms/feet

Scents: lavender, sandalwood, eucalyptus, rose, frankincense, ylang-ylang

Touching Fabrics – Silk, velvet, fleece

Connection with animals

Connection with safe people

Listening to classical music

Breathing as though through a straw

Body scan – Start at the top of your head and slowly become aware of physical sensations as you descend down to your feet. Once identified, what does that body part say? Drawing boundaries / literally

Appropriate touch – define what this is

Movement – Dancing, Rhumba, Pilates

Drawing/painting feelings

Creating a vision board

5 Senses created by Stephanie Covington – looking around identify 5 things you can see, 4 things you can feel, 3 things to hear, 2 things to smell, 1 thing to taste.

12 Step Meetings; CoSa for partners if this feels right to you; SAA, SA for addicts

Writing/ Journaling

Be extra careful.

10 -15 minutes a day to do something enjoyable; not taking care of kids, partner, or other people

"Work" to relax.

Permission to *not* do some things.

Try and keep a healthy structure to focus on things other than the betrayal.

Eating outside. Take your meal and eat in the yard, garden, in a park.

Read Jack Kornfield's meditation for loving-kindness.

Having people say (other than your partner/spouse) that they love you, that you didn't do anything wrong, and they are there for you.

Reading to satiate panic, and then reading as much or little as what is comfortable.

Connecting with plants; digging in dirt, smelling flowers, smelling herb plants.

Lighting candles.

Visualization – wind blowing away - your sadness, putting (whoever is upsetting you) in an ice block and pushing/floating it away

Practicing the Victory Stance by Amy Cuddy

Writing a gratitude list

Touching on the idea "How could this be worse?" to help with perspective.

Do a random act of kindness.

Stay warm – hold onto warm cups with nice warm beverages, sit in the sun, wrap up in warm blankets.

And most of all, be kind to yourself. For addicts, be accountable to others.

Appendix 3

Disclosure Statement

WHAT IS A THERAPEUTIC DISCLOSURE?

We've provided the following as an overview of what to expect with a full therapeutic disclosure. It is by no means meant to be a guide for completing or conducting a disclosure. If you are interested in doing a disclosure, please only do so with a qualified specialist.

Purpose of Disclosure

First and foremost, a full formal disclosure is a transfer of information. Its chief aim is to provide information to the partner of their acting out partner's sexual behaviors. Since secrecy and lies are commonly a core component of sexually addictive behaviors, the disclosure is meant to compile a complete account of the addict's sexual behaviors to the best of his/her knowledge. The process is an opportunity for the addict to be honest with his/her partner and help to restore safety and trust.

The formal disclosure is a facilitated process where the addict relays information to the partner in one place. Rather than doing "staggered" disclosures, which can only compound the traumatic impact of receiving the information, the formal disclosure is a carefully constructed document that the addict prepares and provides to her/his partner.

No longer being in the dark about the nature of the sexual acting out behaviors, lies, and deception that were involved, the addict and partner now share equal footing in the relationship. From this place of equality, the partner is better equipped to make informed decisions about their status in the relationship. Additionally, like cleaning out an infected wound, the disclosure process is an opportunity where an addict and his/her partner can clear out the painful lies in their relationship and come to a renewed place where they can heal.

Ideally, the disclosure is a process used when an addict and a partner are attempting to repair their relationship. The disclosure affords them the best opportunity of starting that process from the foundation of the truth.

What the disclosure IS:
- A transfer of information
- An account of all sexual behaviors
- An opportunity for the addict to bring healing to his/her partner, provide the truth, and begin the possibility of relational restoration.
- An opportunity for the partner to receive information, understand the full nature of her/his partner's sexual acting out behaviors, and to use this knowledge as a way of building safety, healing, and potentially relational restoration.

What the disclosure ISN'T:
- A process where an addict can share some information, while withholding certain information he/she deems too painful for the partner to hear
- An opportunity for a partner to gain further ammunition in divorce/legal proceedings.

Benefits and Risks of Engaging in a Disclosure

Benefits:
- A full disclosure can be a powerfully intimate experience for addicts and partners to come together in truth, perhaps for the first time in their relationship. Intimacy is built through such attributes as honesty, vulnerability, and safety, so the disclosure can be a healing experience for everyone involved. Furthermore, it can provide a foundation upon which a new relationship can be forged.
- Addicts are able to share their secrets, freeing them of the burden of holding those secrets in the relationship.
- Partners are able to receive truth, receive validation for intuition that was undermined, and can thereby begin the process of putting their shattered world together.
- Through the truth, partners are more equipped to make more informed decisions about the relationship
- The relationship has the best opportunity to heal. Just like a festering wound won't heal on its own, by cleaning out the infection of deception, betrayal, and sexual behaviors, the relationship between addict and partner has the possibility of healing and restoration.

Risks:
- Disclosures can be very painful experiences, and are often traumatic in and of themselves
- The partner may hear information that they weren't prepared for, and this can create further trauma symptoms
- The relationship may not be able to be healed after the disclosure.
- Just as in a surgery, things may get "worse before they get better."

Overview of the Disclosure Process

For more information about the specific steps to take to prepare for a therapeutic disclosure, please see a qualified specialist. In general the disclosure will be prepared in three main segments:

- *Pre-disclosure*, where the addict prepares a written document, tailored to the information requested from the partner, and also where both addict and partner prepare for the disclosure session and the immediate days following the disclosure
- *Disclosure*, where the disclosure document is read and processed in a safe space. This should be established ahead of time and given preference to where the partner feels safest.
- *Post-disclosure*, where the addict and partner make a plan for the time post-disclosure as well as safety boundaries to be implemented post-disclosure.

Please note: every disclosure is unique since every individual and every relationship is unique.

Appendix 4

Sexual Addiction and Recovery - Eight Stages of Grief

Sexual addiction often leaves broken relationships in its wake. For spouses living or in relationship with a sex addict, dealing with the grieving process requires a great deal of effort. It also requires understanding the various stages of grief so that when the spouse is dealing with the recovery process, there will be fewer surprises.

Below are the extended stages of grief in a **sex addiction recovery** process. Also, for the addict, they experience tremendous loss as well. Because we now know the addiction covers repressed emotions, anything buried begins to surface to be acknowledged and processed.

Shock and Denial
In this stage, the partner suffers from shock on knowing she has suffered a great wound. Shock acts to defend the mind. When we are in shock we may deny facts that have actually happened. A person in grief may feel she is dreaming and that she cannot accept the situation. Simple tasks and decisions often are not carried out or not executed well by a person in shock.

For the addict, he also is in shock that his two worlds have collided and secrets he would have never shared are now known. There is a lot of denial as to the depth and extent of the acting out behaviors. There also can be denial that this actually has crossed a line into addiction. He, also, becomes foggy and disoriented, sometimes having difficulty at work and/or completing daily tasks and commitments.

Pain and Guilt

At this stage, the grieving person realizes that the loss that has happened is true. This is the most chaotic and scary stage of grief. Many partners start to use alcohol and drugs at this stage. Partners may feel guilt or remorse for being in the relationship or having children with this person, even though they love their kids deeply. Sometimes, in grief, partners blame themselves and consider themselves responsible for the addiction and the resulting losses.

For the addict, most experience deep remorse and pain for the consequences occurring. They, too, may use spending money, drugs or alcohol to try and remediate the pain. Because of the lack of practice with expressing feelings, they may only have "I'm sorry" as a response to the partner's pain. Or they may go numb or silent.

Anger

The next stage is anger. The partner may get angry due to the injustice that has happened to her or she may get angry with the person responsible for the loss in her life. This, often, can turn to rage. Although anger is justifiable, it often is unproductive in the relationship. Finding ways to discharge the rage, be able to articulate the underlying feelings and have the addict mirror and take ownership is key.

The addict, although many feel he doesn't deserve to feel angry, does! Mainly, he is angry at himself, but this often gets expressed as anger towards his partner, society, or women in general. He may also get angry and frustrated with questions and probes into his recovery process. This, although a natural part of grieving, is also unproductive in the relationship. Finding new ways to work with this intense emotion is important.

Bargaining

After the painful stage of anger, the partner in grief gets frustrated and may try to compensate for the loss. Some people try to regain a sense of control over the addict, their children, their finances, etc. There may be a move to revert back to old relationship dynamics and to try and compensate for what has been lost. Partners at this stage almost always consider staying in the relationship, and leaving. Addicts can misunderstand and start moving to separate. It is wise to understand this is part of the process. We can't guarantee that in the Acceptance stage there will not be a divorce and unless she removes her rings and files for divorce, we are not there yet.

For the addict, he will do all kinds of bargaining. This can include spending less time at meetings and "more time with the family". He may begin to buy gifts or try to console the partner in different ways. He may want to offer more information about his acting out (which is why we suggest a Disclosure soon after Discovery). He also may consider leaving and staying in the marriage. We know addicts have a stronger fight or flight response, so we do not encourage the addict initiating separation or divorce at this stage.

Depression and Sorrow

Here the partner accepts the loss but is unable to cope with it. Depressed and demoralized, the person is in despair and behaves passively. She sees no remedy to the loss and can feel hopeless regarding staying in the relationship or leaving and ever finding someone else as a partner. Sadness can lead to depression at this stage.

The addict can experience a hopeless, flat feeling. If he is in recovery, he may feel he has tried so hard but cannot "fix" his partner's pain, anger, and sadness. He also feels demoralized. There are times where we need to watch for suicidal ideation.

Testing and Reconstruction
This is the testing stage in which the sad or depressed partner starts to engage in other activities so as to minimalize the disturbing sorrow. For the first time she realizes she is going to survive. This is the beginning of the next and last stage: acceptance. Here, she starts the process of reconstructing her life. Slowly, she starts to come back to life.

He realizes that whatever the outcome of his relationship, he will be okay. Many times this is when the addict does recovery for himself instead of for his partner or children. There is a calmness and acceptance to life in general, versus frustration and anxiety.

Acceptance
This is the final stage of the seven stages of grief, when the grieving partner accepts reality. This reality is that her partner is indeed a sex addict and not just a jerk. She becomes stable as a separate unique person from the addict. Acceptance stage creates hope and the partner starts believing in herself. She does not blame or take responsibility for the addict. Reality and facts of life are accepted and she moves forward in her life.

The addict finds peace in knowing he is doing the very best he can to be sober and understand the roots and the addiction and get help and support. He does not have to hide behind old coping skills to defend, minimalize, fabricate or lie about what he does or who he is. Most of all, he can accept he is not perfect and that he makes mistakes but can take responsibility and make mature leveled decisions in life.

Appendix 5

PATHOS

PATHOS is a brief assessment of sexual addiction derived from the Sexual Addiction Screening Test (SAST) developed by Patrick Carnes et al. The PATHOS assessment helps clinicians to determine whether or not sex addiction treatment is appropriate for the client/patient

In a 2012 study headed by Dr. Patrick Carnes* it was estimated that sexual addiction is estimated to afflict up to 3% to 6% of the population. However, many clinicians lack clear criteria for detecting potential cases.

PATHOS is a brief sexual addiction screening questionnaire. The aforementioned clinical study from Carnes, et. al., found PATHOS as clinically significant for effectively classifying patient's appropriateness for entering treatment as potential sex addicts.

*Carnes PJ, Green BA, Merlo LJ, Polles A, Carnes S, Gold MS, March 6, 2012 (1):29-34. PATHOS: a brief screening application for assessing sexual addiction. doi: 10.1097/ADM.0b013e3182251a28.

PATHOS stands for the six assessment questions:

Preoccupied – Do you often find yourself preoccupied with sexual thoughts?

Ashamed – Do you hide some of your sexual behavior from others?

Treatment – Have you ever sought therapy for sexual behavior you did not like?

Hurt others – Has anyone been hurt emotionally because of your sexual behavior?

Out of control – Do you feel controlled by your sexual desire?

Sad – When you have sex, do you feel depressed afterwards?

A positive response to just one of the six questions would indicate a need for additional assessment with a certified sex addiction therapist (CSAT).
Two or more positive responses are considered a strong indication that treatment is needed.

180

Where to go for help

12 Step Programs are a cornerstone of breaking free from compulsive behavior.

For sex addiction you can find meetings at …
Sexaholics Anonymous (SA)
www.sa.org
866-424-8777

Sex Addicts Anonymous (SAA)
www.saa-recovery.org
800-477-8191

Sex and Love Addicts Anonymous (SLAA)
www.slaafws.org
210-828-7900

Faith-based sex addiction meetings …

Pure Desire
www.puredesire.org/en/

Guard Your Eyes
guardyoureyes.com/

XXX Church
www.xxxchurch.com/

Celebrate Recovery
www.celebraterecovery.com/

L.I.F.E. Groups
http://www.freedomeveryday.org/

For alcoholism...
Alcoholics Anonymous (AA)
www.aa.org
212-870-3400

For drug addiction....
Narcotics Anonymous
www.na.org
818-773-9999

Marijuana Anonymous
www.marijuana-anonymous.org
800-766-6779

Crystal Meth Anonymous
www.crystalmeth.org

For support if your spouse is addicted to sex or porn

The Association of Partners of Sex Addicts Trauma
Specialists (APSATS)
www.apsats.org
(513) 644-8023

Partners of Sex Addicts Resource Center
www.posarc.com

Partners of Sex Addicts (PoSA) Meetings
www.posarc.com/healing-support-main/posa-meetings

Women in the Battle Workshops (Faith-based workshops
for betrayed spouses)
newlife.com/workshops/restore-intensive-workshop/

If you ascribe to a 12-step perspective on healing from
betrayal trauma:
Codependents of sex addicts (COSA)
www.cosa-recovery.org
763-537-6904

S-Anon
www.sanon.org
800-210-8141

If you are both accessing 12 step programs:

Recovering Couples Anonymous (RCA)
www.recovering-couples.org
510-663-2312

Additional Resources

A.A. Big Book by The Augustine Fellowship, Sex & Love Addicts Anonymous

As We Understood by Al-Anon

Courage to Change by Al-Anon

One Day at a Time in Al-Anon by Al-Anon

Opening Our Hearts; Transforming Our Losses by Al-Anon

Reflections of Hope by S-Anon

S-Anon Twelve Steps by S-Anon

Working the S-Anon Program by S-Anon

The White Book by Sexaholics Anonymous

The Green Book by Sex Addicts Anonymous

S.L.A.A.

Helping her Heal video by Doug Weiss

If you would like to have more information about sex addiction the following books can be helpful:

Books Regarding Trauma

Waking The Tiger
Peter Levine
Waking the Tiger normalizes the symptoms of trauma and the steps needed to heal them. The reader is taken on a guided tour of the subtle, yet powerful impulses that govern our responses to overwhelming life events. To do this, it employs a series of exercises that help us focus on bodily sensations. Through heightened awareness of these sensations trauma can be healed.

The Trauma Spectrum
Robert Scaer
Our experiences of trauma sow the seeds of many persistent and misunderstood medical problems such as chronic fatigue syndrome and various maladies of the immune system. Because of our inadequate understanding of the relationship of mind and body in processing these traumas, many of us suffer needlessly from our exposure to life's traumas. Robert Scaer offers hope to those who wish to transform trauma and better understand their lives.

BrainSpotting: The Revolutionary New Therapy for Rapid and Effective Change
David Grand
"Brainspotting lets the therapist and client participate together in the healing process," explains Dr. Grand. "It allows us to harness the brain's natural ability for self-scanning, so we can activate, locate, and process the sources of trauma and distress in the body." With Brainspotting, this pioneering researcher

introduces an invaluable tool that can support virtually any form
of therapeutic practice and greatly accelerate our ability to heal.

*Getting Past Your Past: Take Control of Your Life with Self-Help
Techniques from EMDR Therapy*
Francine Shapiro
Whether we've experienced small setbacks or major traumas, we
are all influenced by memories and experiences we may not
remember or don't fully understand. Getting Past Your Past
offers practical procedures that demystify the human condition
and empower readers looking to achieve real change. Shapiro,
the creator of EMDR (Eye Movement Desensitization and
Reprocessing), explains how our personalities develop and why
we become trapped into feeling, believing and acting in ways
that don't serve us. Through detailed examples and exercises
readers will learn to understand themselves, and why the people
in their lives act the way they do. Most importantly, readers will
also learn techniques to improve their relationships, break
through emotional barriers, overcome limitations and excel in
ways taught to Olympic athletes, successful executives and
performers. An easy conversational style, humor and fascinating
real life stories make it simple to understand the brain science,
why we get stuck in various ways and what to do about it.

Books for Partners of Sex Addicts

Your Sexually Addicted Spouse: How Partners Can Cope and Heal
Barbara Steffens, Marsha Means
The authors lay out the case that 12 step programs for partners of sex addicts can be harmful in labeling the partner as a co-addict, or co-dependent, and that the pain that partners experience after discovery of their partner's behavior is best understood as a trauma that can have long lasting effects.

Mending A Shattered Heart: A Guide for Partners of Sex Addicts
Stephanie Carnes, Ph.D.
A go-to guide covering important subjects such as whether to stay in the relationship or leave, when and how life gets better, how to set boundaries and what to say to the children.

Back From Betrayal: Recovering From His Affairs, Third Edition
Jennifer P. Schneider
This is a new edition of a classic book for women and men whose spouses or partners have had multiple affairs or sex addiction problems. Dr. Schneider explains how Twelve Step recovery programs can work for you, and provides straightforward guidance on how to find self-help groups and how to choose a therapist. The 2005 Third Edition is expanded and updated, with additional material for men whose partners have affairs, a chapter on cybersex and Internet affairs, information on disclosing secrets to one's partner and children, and updated medical information on sexually transmitted diseases.

Ready to Heal
Kelly McDaniel
Help for those struggling in a relationship with a sex addict, facing their own sex addiction, obsessing about someone who

doesn't want you, or looking for deeper understanding of romantic patterns. At its core, love and sex addiction is a longing for intimacy. Since love, connection, and sexual intimacy are basic human needs, healing addictive relationships prepares you to give and receive love in healthy ways. Part of being ready to heal is having faith that, although you don't know what will happen, you are prepared to move forward on the journey.

Letters To A Sex Addict: The Journey through Grief and Betrayal
Wendy Conquest
This collection of fictional letters, inspired by real life, viscerally expresses what the partner of a sex addict is thinking and feeling. Readers will resonate with the emotional and psychological strain as well as grasp the hope that, with help, this disaster can be overcome.

Facing Heartbreak: Steps to Recovery for Partners of Sex Addicts
Stefanie Carnes, Mari A. Lee, Anthony D. Rodriguez
When you discover that the person you loved and trusted most in the world is hiding a secret life as a sex addict, the result can be devastating. Facing that heartbreak is what this book is all about. The healing process will take time regardless of whether you decide to stay in the relationship or leave. Facing Heartbreak weaves real life stories with practical therapeutic advice and specific tasks that gently educate, empower, and guide the partner of the sex addict through a process of recovery.

Sex Addiction: The Partner's Perspective: A Comprehensive Guide to Understanding and Surviving Sex Addiction for Partners and Those who Want to Help Them
Paula Hall
This book serves as a guide for partners of sex addicts and

those who want to help them to establish stability and control in their lives. It has been written with facts and exercises in such a way to help partners navigate through the shock of discovery and empowering them to make decisions for their future. Survey data helps inform the empowering exercises in the book.

Spouses of Sex Addicts: Hope for the Journey
Francoise Mastroianni and Richard Blankenship
This book has been written using the stories of many spouses who have navigated their way through the darkness of the night and into the light of hope and healing. Spouses of Sex Addicts is a continuation of S.A.R.A.H. (Spouses of Addicts Rebuilding and Healing.) It includes updated stories, more emphasis on healing from trauma, and information on working with children who have been exposed to sexual addiction. This book also has a companion workbook.

Books about Sex Addiction

Don't Call It Love: Recovery from Sexual Addiction
Patrick Carnes, Ph.D.
Based on the candid testimony of more than one thousand recovering sex addicts in the first major scientific study of the disorder, this book includes the findings of Carnes' research. It also has advice from the addicts and partners of sex addicts involved in the study.

Understanding and Treating Sex Addiction: A comprehensive guide for people who struggle with sex addiction and those who want to help them
Paula Hall
This work explains why an increasing number of people are inadvertently finding their lives devastated by their sexual behaviors. It explores the latest scientific understandings and research into why pornography, cybersex, visiting sex workers, fetishes and multiple affairs can come to control some people's lives to the point that they can't stop. It explains how sex addiction is not a moral issue, as some assume, but a health issue that we as a society need to start taking seriously.

Naked in Public: A Memoir of Recovery from Sex Addiction and Other Temporary Insanities
Staci Sprout
In this intensely personal memoir, the author offers a vulnerable account of her recovery journey from the painful world of sexual intrigue and addiction.

In the Shadows of the Net: Breaking Free of Compulsive Online Sexual Behavior
Patrick Carnes, David Delmonico, and Elizabeth Griffin.
As Internet usage has exploded in recent years, so has the

prevalence of compulsive online sexual behavior. This second edition is updated with the latest information, equipping readers with specific strategies for recognizing and changing compulsive sexual behaviors.

Cruise Control: Understanding Sex Addiction in Gay Men
Robert Weiss.
Avoiding political and moral arguments this book focuses on the clinical approach, asking the question, "Is your sexual behavior causing problems in other areas of your life?" *Cruise Control* leads men to a better understanding of the difference between sexual compulsion and non-addictive sexual behavior within the gay experience, and it explains what resources are available for recovery.

The Porn Trap: The Essential Guide To Overcoming Problems Caused By Pornography
Wendy Maltz and Larry Maltz
In this recovery guide, sex and relationship therapists Wendy and Larry Maltz shed new light on the compelling nature and destructive power of today's instantly available pornography.

Untangling the Web
Jennifer Schneider and Robert Weiss
With personal stories from addicts and their significant others, this updated resource offers realistic healing strategies for anyone experiencing the devastating impact of Internet pornography and sex addiction on intimacy, relationships, career, health, and self-respect.

Confronting Pornography: A Guide to Prevention and Recovery for
Individuals, Loved Ones, and Leaders
Mark D. Chamberlain
A collection of articles from professional counselors, leaders, and individuals who have dealt with pornography problems personally, this useful book is an invaluable resource. It offers understanding, powerful tools based in gospel principles, and, most of all, hope.

Connection and Healing: A 200-Day Journey into Recovery
Russ Pope and Dan Green
This unique journal is designed to help recovering addicts to express themselves in a positive way by offering daily meditations for inspiration as well as help in identifying the various emotions that are felt each day.

When He's Married to Mom: How to Help Mother-Enmeshed Men
Open Their Hearts to True Love and Commitment
Ken Adams
Clinical psychologist and renowned intimacy expert Adams goes beyond the stereotypes of momma's boys and meddling mothers to explain how mother-son enmeshment affects everyone: the mother, the son, and the woman who loves him.

Worthy of her Trust: What You Need to Do to Rebuild Sexual Integrity
and Win Her Back
Stephen Arterburn and Jason Martinkus
This faith-based book serves as a guide through the process of rebuilding relationships after betrayal. It addresses how to be truly transparent, building safety around triggers and temptations, developing trust-building strategies, exploring forgiveness and restitution, and creating an Amends Matrix. This book also provides encouragement to betrayed partners.

Pure Desire: How One Man's Triumph Can Help Others Break Free from Sexual Temptation
Ted Roberts
In this faith-based book, Dr. Roberts shares hope for breaking free from sexual bondage. Using his personal journey as well as practical guidance, he provides a map for walking in victory.

Pure Eyes: A Man's Guide to Sexual Integrity
Craig Gross and Steven Luff
This book takes a faith-based easy-to-use approach for building wholeness in the lives of men struggling with addiction to pornography. Gross and Luff provide this book as a resource to help men end the cycle of self-hatred, shame and embarrassment in using pornography.

Your Brain on Porn: Internet Pornography and the Emerging Science of Addiction
Gary Wilson
In this book, Gary Wilson provides a concise introduction to the phenomenon of internet porn addiction that draws on both first-person accounts and the findings of cognitive neuroscience. In a voice that is generous and humane, he also offers advice for those who want to stop using internet pornography. The publication of Your Brain on Porn is a landmark in our attempts to understand, and remain balanced in, a world where addiction is big business.

Sex Addiction as Affect Dysregulation: A Neurobiologically Informed Holistic Treatment
Alexandra Katehakis
This book integrates cutting-edge research, case studies, and patient records to explicate neurophysiological, psychological, and cultural forces priming and maintaining sex addiction. Katehakis uses this integration to detail her Psychobiological

Approach to Sex Addiction Treatment (PASAT) – an approach that restores patients' interpersonal, sexual, and spiritual relationality.

For Love and Money: Exploring Sexual and Financial Betrayal in Relationship
Debra Kaplan
This book turns a provocative, literary lens on the worlds of sex, money and relational power. It delivers an unparalleled and cutting-edge perspective about sexual, financial and relational exploitation from Wall Street to Main Street; boardroom to bedroom. This exploration merges academic investigation, therapeutic narrative and case study. It is a ground breaking must read for those individuals interested in restoring sexual and financial health to their lives.

Acknowledgments

We would, together, like to acknowledge our esteemed colleagues who have generously read and given us feedback for our book, especially Barb Steffens, Stefanie Carnes, Mari Lee, Ken Adams, Rob Weiss, Deb Kaplan, Carol Juergensen Sheets, Richard Blankenship, Ted Roberts, Dorit Reichental, Sheri Keffer, Jes Montgomery, Todd Love, and Sam Alibrando.

To our clients over the years, we honor each and every step you've taken towards recovery, healing from trauma, and restoring relationships. Thank you for letting us journey on the road with you – your experience, strength, and hope have made this book possible.

Marianne Harkin, thank you for editing our book and taking it to the next level. And Violet Farley, thank you for your creative inspiration for the cover art.

And to all the men, women, couples, and families who are doing the work of recovery one day at a time, thank you for inspiring us each and every day. YOU CAN DO THIS!

From Dan:

First and foremost I would like to acknowledge my wife, who has championed me in this project and in my passion to work with men and women impacted by sex addiction. Thanks for always spurring me on to keep growing professionally and personally. You are an inspiration – I couldn't do this without you!

Wendy, I'm grateful for our collaboration and friendship that has grown week after week on this book. You are a truly gifted writer and clinician.

To my amazing friends, family, and colleagues, thank you for believing in me and helping me grow into the therapist and human being that I am today. You are too many to name here, but a few who especially made this book happen: Seth, Julia, Peter, Adam, Stephanie, Ed, Diane, Dorit Reichental, Janice Caudill, Barb Steffens, Heather, Juan Carlos, Dairek, and Joanna. Thank you from the bottom of my heart.

There are many who have been trudging the road of happy destiny with me, too many to list here. But I especially want to acknowledge Sam A, RK, SC, DM, DP, SH, SGK, SL, SC, JK, JG, JL, JVS, and JH. Thank you all for helping make the promises come true for me one day at a time.

From Wendy:

To Dan Drake, who without his courage, dedication, selflessness, amazing insight and writing ability, this book would not be. Thank you Dan. I couldn't ask for a better writing partner.

Dan's wife, Kari, has played a major part, keeping us on track, being an artistic partner and a constant encouraging friend. Thank you Kari.

Therapists in my world who are always there for me. By name, Nora Swan Foster, Cynthia Ropek, Dan Baur, Kristy Howlett, Jill Krush, and Craig Revord.

A special thank you to Gary Allen for his constant wide and benevolent presence.

There are many friends who are there for me constantly including Chris Thatcher, Jane Saltzman, Joan and Russ Game, Eli Ackerstein, Christine Hurley, Belle Schmidt, Barbara Hoffman and Brenna Hopkins.

Finally, I'd like to thank my mother who died shortly before publication. Irene Benno instilled in me the belief that anything is possible and to always follow your dreams. With her gone, Ted Atz has stepped in being perpetually positive and encouraging. I am so grateful.

About the Authors

Wendy Conquest is a Licensed Professional Counselor, certified sex addiction therapist and supervisor (CSAT-S). She is also certified in Integrative Body Psychotherapy and Brainspotting, trained in EMDR and equine assisted therapy. She specializes in and has extensive experience working with trauma, sexual abuse, and healthy sexuality.

Wendy is the author of *Letters To A Sex Addict; the Journey through Grief and Betrayal.* She is also the Founder and President of SACC Corp., in Boulder, Colorado, an organization that is dedicated to treating sex addiction and teaching healthy sexuality.

Dan Drake is a licensed therapist in Los Angeles, California. He is a Certified Sex Addiction Therapist Supervisor, a Certified Clinical Partner Specialist, and he is EMDR trained. He has received two post doctorate degrees from Fuller Theological seminary in Marital and Family Therapy and in Theology.

Dan uses his training and specializations to treat sex addicts, their partners, and families in his group practice. In addition to his clinical background, he has taught and spoken domestically and internationally. His passion is to help his clients restore relational, mental, emotional, physical, and spiritual wholeness to their lives.

Made in the USA
Middletown, DE
20 June 2017